Polycystic Ovarian Syndrome

Edited by Zhengchao Wang

Published in London, United Kingdom

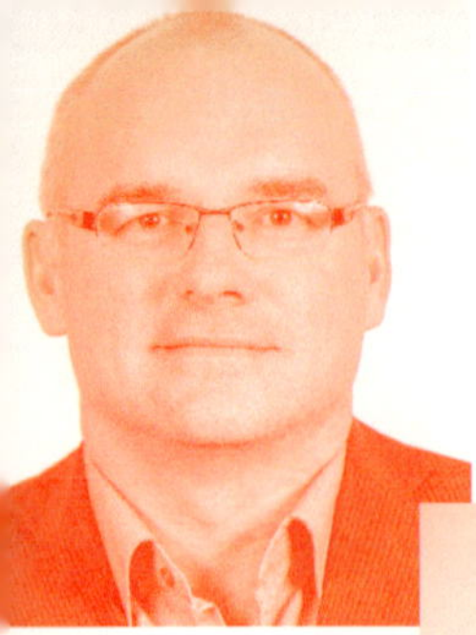
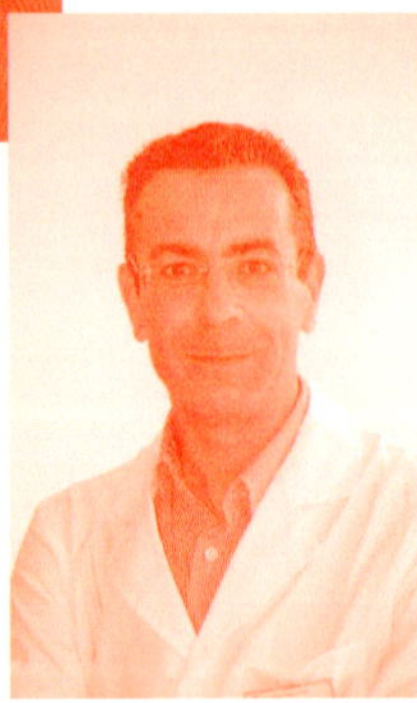
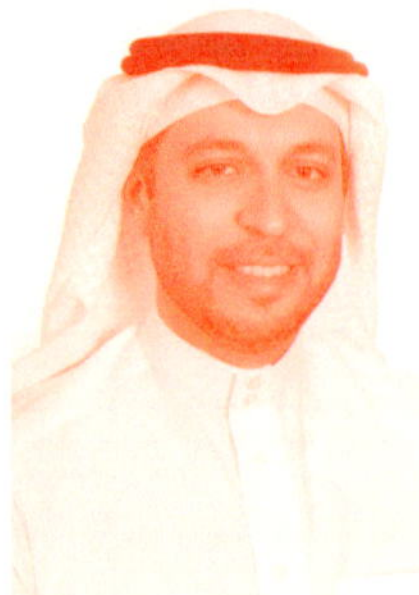
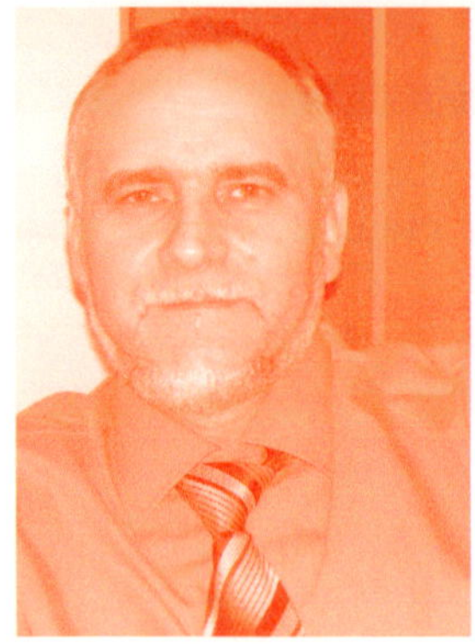
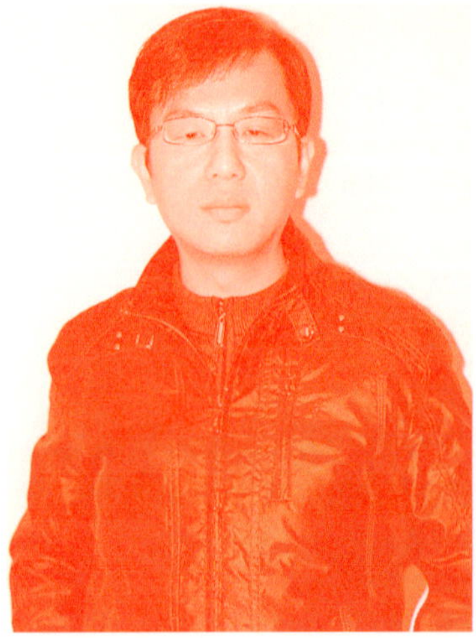
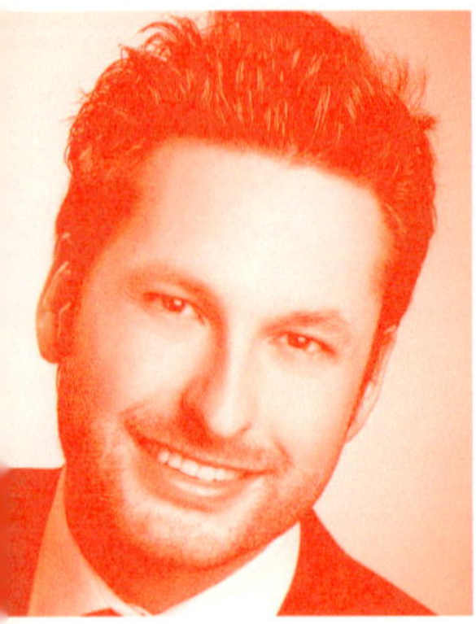
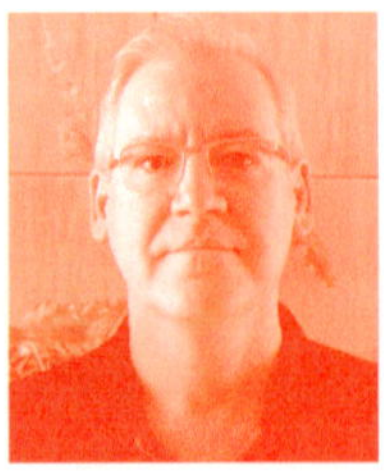

IntechOpen

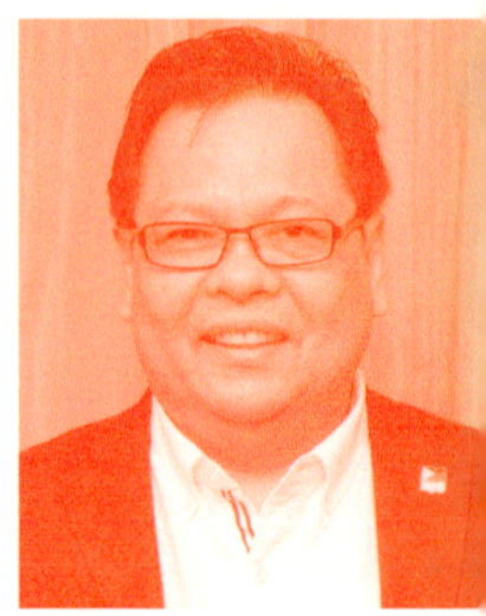
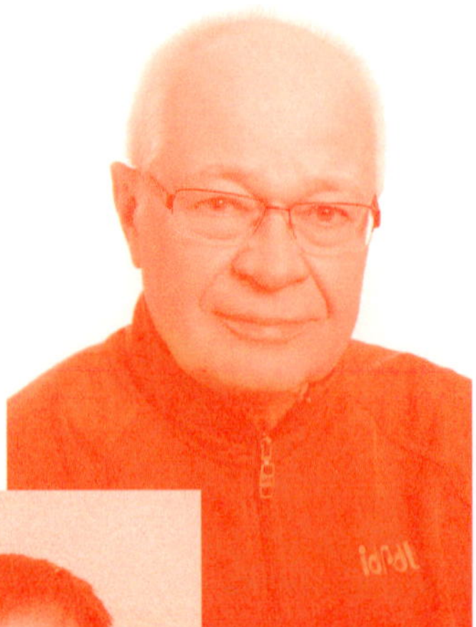
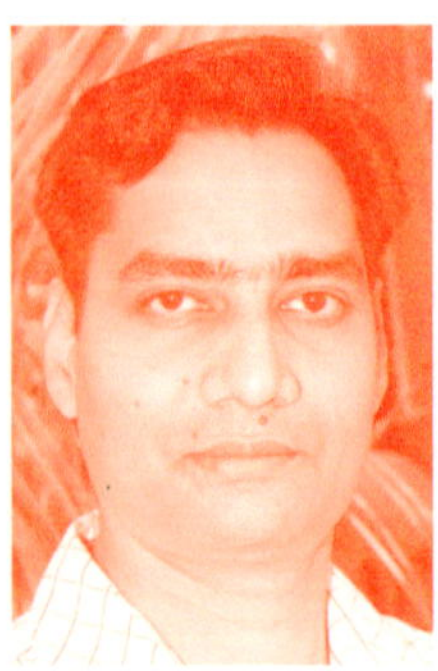
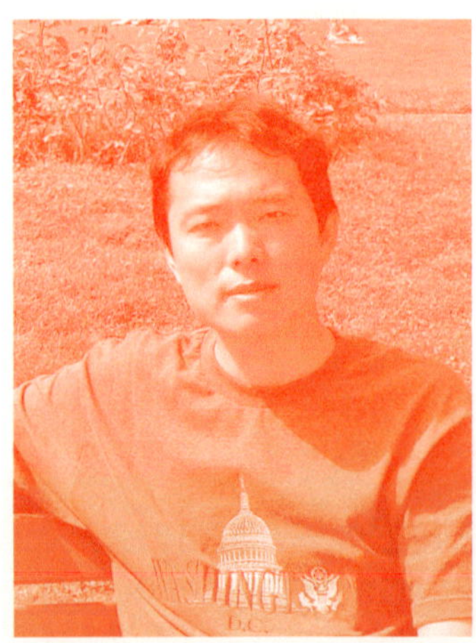
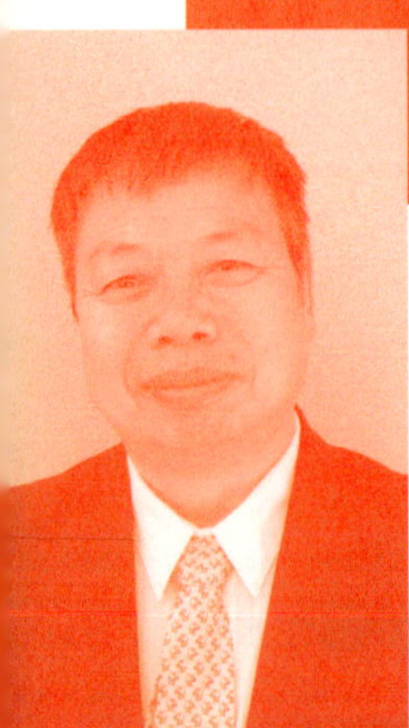
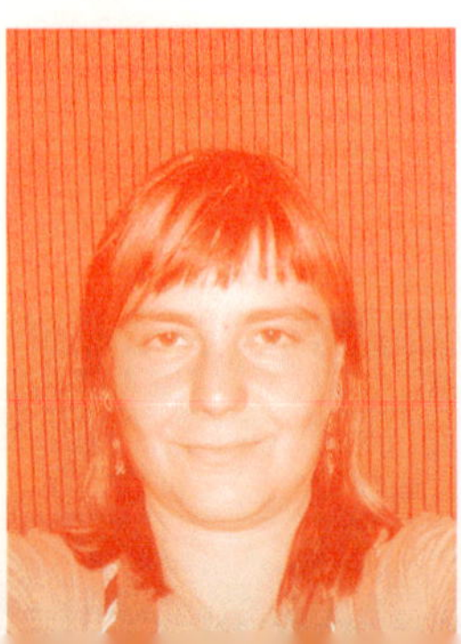

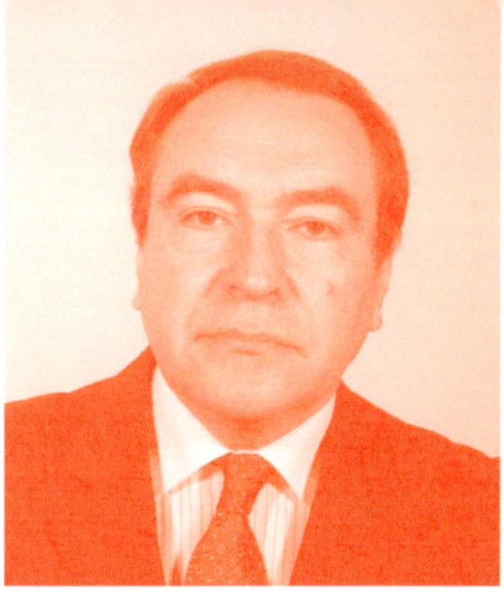
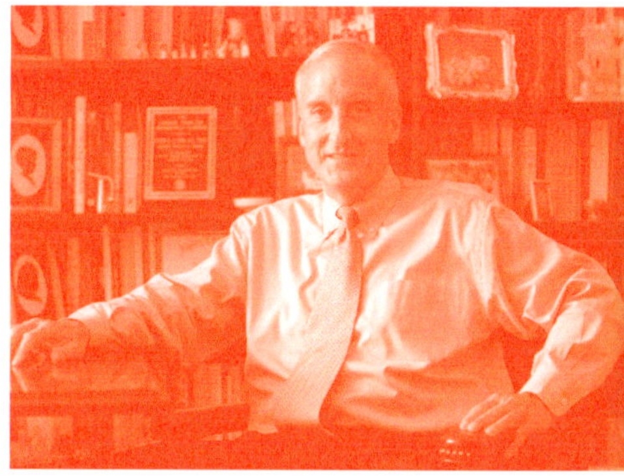
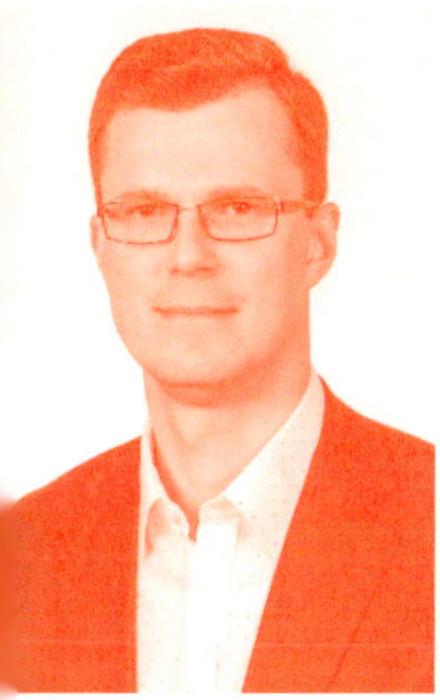
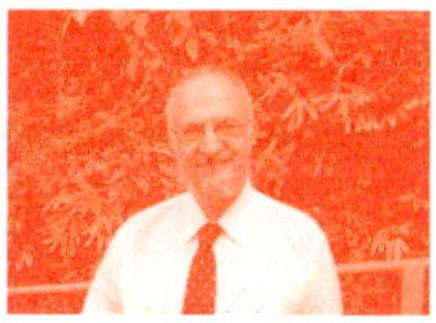
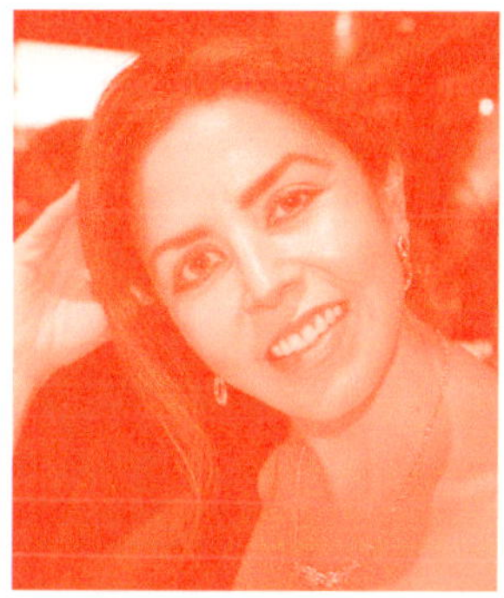

Supporting open minds since 2005

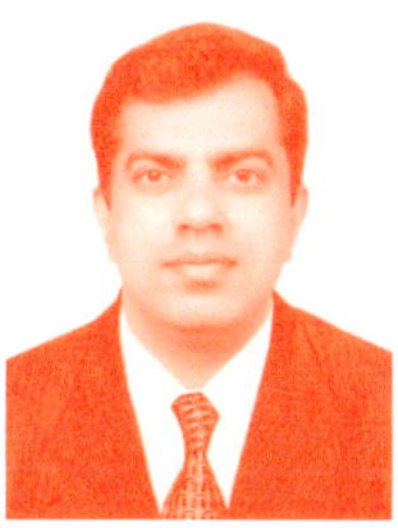
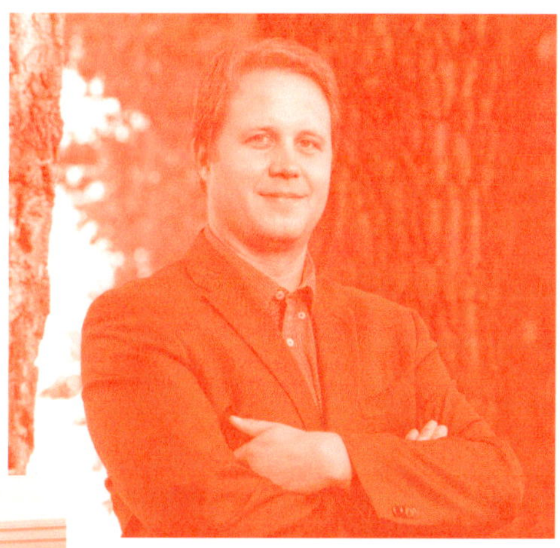
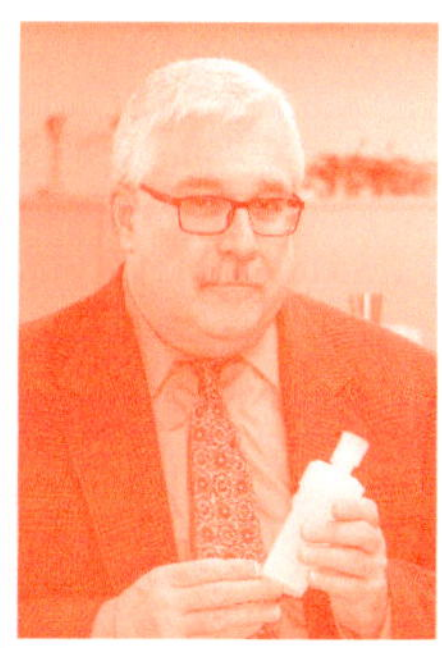
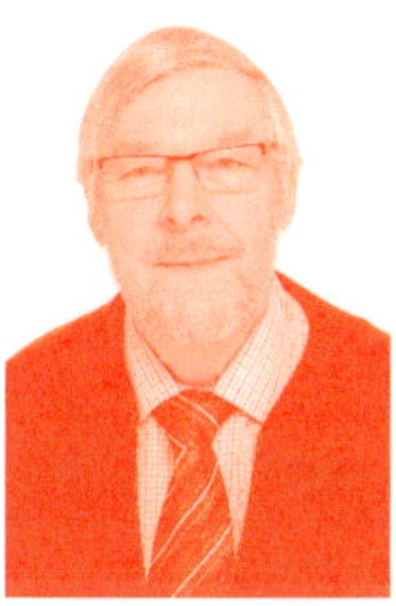
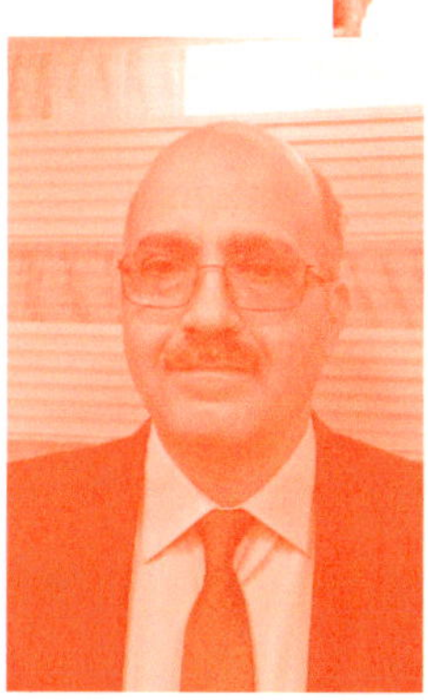
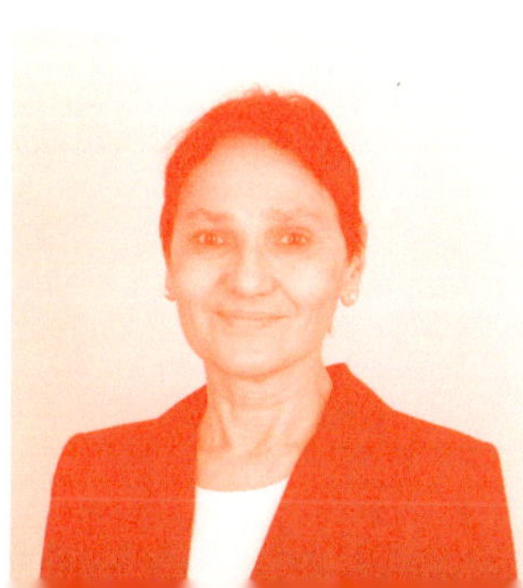
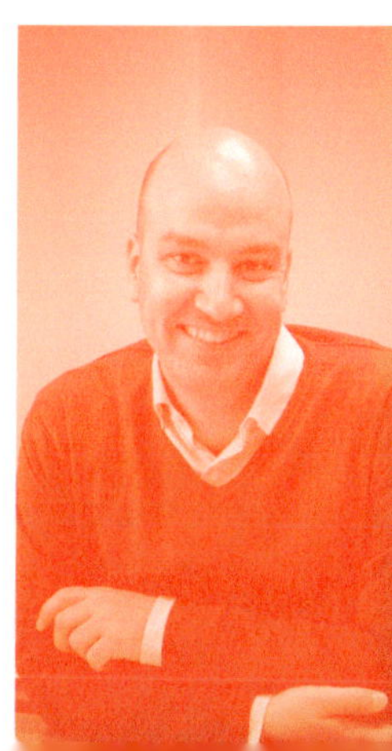

Polycystic Ovarian Syndrome
http://dx.doi.org/10.5772/intechopen.83161
Edited by Zhengchao Wang

Contributors
Bassim Alsadi, Wang Fan, Yu Zhen, Chen Gang, Han Junyong, Shaobing Wang, Zhenghong Zhang, Yiping Liu, Yan Zhang, Zhengchao Wang, Fengping Lin, Qingqiang Lin, Hong Zhang, Jiuhua Zhao, Zeti-Azura Mohamed-Hussein, Nor Afiqah-Aleng, Vita Dolžan, Rok Herman, Mojca Jensterle Sever, Andrej Janež, Maria Mitkova Orbetzova, Hassan S Abduljabbar

First published in London, United Kingdom, 2020 by IntechOpen
IntechOpen is the global imprint of INTECHOPEN LIMITED, registered in England and Wales, registration number: 11086078, 7th floor, 10 Lower Thames Street, London, EC3R 6AF, United Kingdom
Printed in Croatia

British Library Cataloguing-in-Publication Data
A catalogue record for this book is available from the British Library

Additional hard and PDF copies can be obtained from orders@intechopen.com

Polycystic Ovarian Syndrome
Edited by Zhengchao Wang
p. cm.
Print ISBN 978-1-83880-289-9
Online ISBN 978-1-83880-290-5
eBook (PDF) ISBN 978-1-83880-415-2

Meet the editor

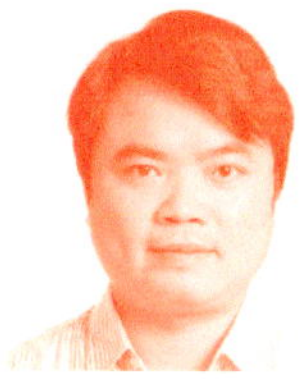

Dr Zhengchao Wang is a full professor at the College of Life Sciences, Fujian Normal University (China). He is a Principal Investigator for General Program for National Natural Science Foundation of China and Program for New Century Excellent Talents in University of Ministry of Education of China. He is also a team leader in the Fujian Provincial Key Laboratory for Developmental Biology and Neurosciences, Key Laboratory of Optoelectronic Science and Technology for Medicine of Ministry of Education. He obtained his PhD in 2008 and has a long teaching and research career. He has published 161 scientific papers in English or Chinese, participated in approximately 30 grants, and published 11 books as the editor in his specialty and related diseases.

Contents

Preface XI

Section 1
Clinical Features of Polycystic Ovarian Syndrome 1

Chapter 1 3
Clinical Features of PCOS
by Bassim Alsadi

Chapter 2 17
Clinical Impact of Insulin Resistance in Women with Polycystic Ovary Syndrome
by Maria Mitkova Orbetzova

Chapter 3 47
Effects of Exercise Intervention on the Improvement of Polycystic Ovary Syndrome
by Shaobing Wang, Zhenghong Zhang and Yiping Liu

Chapter 4 63
Effect of Aromatase Inhibitors versus Clomiphene Citrate for Ovulation Induction in Infertile Women with Ovulatory Dysfunction (PCO)
by Hassan S.O. Abduljabbar, Magda Hagras and Rania Magadmy

Section 2
Basic Researches of Polycystic Ovary Syndrome 71

Chapter 5 73
Endocrine Characteristics and Regulatory Mechanism of Follicular Development and Ovulation Failure in Mammalian Ovary
by Zhenghong Zhang, Yan Zhang, Fengping Lin and Zhengchao Wang

Chapter 6 85
Expression and Contribution of Insulin Signaling Pathway to the Development of Polycystic Ovary Syndrome
by Qingqiang Lin, Hong Zhang, Jiuhua Zhao and Zhengchao Wang

Chapter 7 95
Roles of ncRNAs in Ovarian Dysfunction of Polycystic Ovary Syndrome
by Junyong Han, Zhen Yu, Gang Chen and Fan Wang

Chapter 8 105
Interplay between Oxidative Stress and Chronic Inflammation in PCOS: The Role of Genetic Variability in PCOS Risk and Treatment Responses
by Rok Herman, Mojca Jensterle Sever, Andrej Janež and Vita Dolžan

Chapter 9 125
Computational Systems Analysis on Polycystic Ovarian Syndrome (PCOS)
by Nor Afiqah-Aleng and Zeti-Azura Mohamed-Hussein

Preface

Polycystic ovary syndrome (PCOS) is a major health problem with a heterogeneous hormone-imbalance disorder that occurs in approximately 4~18% of reproductive-aged women worldwide, which is characterized by hyperandrogenism, ovulatory process dysfunction, and polycystic ovaries.

PCOS is affected by various factors and there are no unique diagnostic criteria in different regions, due to the heterogeneity of clinical manifestations and endocrine system changes of PCOS. Therefore, it is often difficult to accurately diagnose women with PCOS, as the signs and symptoms of PCOS can vary among individuals. Although PCOS is usually diagnosed during the early reproductive years, the precise pathogenesis of PCOS remains unclear. An increasing number of studies have demonstrated that the insulin signaling pathway has an important role in the pathophysiology of PCOS, including phosphatidylinositol 3-kinase and protein kinase B signaling, which is critically implicated in insulin resistance, androgen secretion, obesity, and follicular development. PCOS manifests as defective ovarian steroid biosynthesis and hyperandrogenemia, and 50~70% of women with PCOS exhibit insulin resistance and are hyperinsulinemic, indicating that insulin resistance and hyperinsulinism may have an important role in the pathophysiology of PCOS.

This book intends to provide the reader with a comprehensive overview of the latest PCOS research and to benefit the population of women with PCOS. At last, it is my hope that this book is meaningful to the clinicians who care for women with PCOS and to the researchers who investigate the complexities of this disorder.

Dr. Zhengchao Wang
Provincial Key Laboratory for Developmental Biology and Neurosciences,
College of Life Sciences,
Fujian Normal University,
Fuzhou, China

Section 1

Clinical Features of Polycystic Ovarian Syndrome

Chapter 1

Clinical Features of PCOS

Bassim Alsadi

Abstract

Polycystic ovary syndrome (PCOS) is a widespread pathology that affects multiple aspects of the general health of women, with long-term effects that go well beyond the reproductive age. The considerable variability of the clinical presentation, together with the lack of universally accepted diagnostic criteria, has so far contributed to making it difficult to identify a clear etiology of the disease. The exact etiology of PCOS is still not perfectly clear to date. It is therefore a multifactorial etiology, sharing of genetic and environmental factors. The contribution of genetics to the pathogenesis of PCOS is not due to a single gene but inheritance of gene clusters. The term "polycystic ovary syndrome" does not completely reflect the complexity of this syndrome which manifests a wide spectrum of clinical manifestations and comorbidity and important metabolic implications. PCOS patients showed an increase risk of developing type 2 diabetes mellitus, dyslipidaemia, endometrial cancer and cardiovascular diseases. The clinical aspects of PCOS are hyperandrogenism, oligomenorrhoea and ultrasound morphology of the ovary. The identification of the different manifestations of PCOS in the various phases of life, can, of course, help to organize individual therapeutic strategies and likely to prevent long-term metabolic consequences. The therapeutic choices will be based on the type and extent of the disorders and if there is a desire for pregnancy.

Keywords: polycystic ovary syndrome, hyperandrogenism, ultrasound, insulin, insulin resistance, metformin, hyperinsulinaemia, inositol, infertility, menstrual irregularities, anovulation, obesity

1. Introduction

Polycystic ovary syndrome (PCOS) was first observed by Stein and Leventhal who in 1935 described seven women with amenorrhoea, hirsutism and increased volume of the ovaries characterized by the presence of numerous cysts [1]. The exact etiology of PCOS is still not perfectly clear to date. It is therefore a multifactorial etiology, sharing of genetic and environmental factors [2]. The contribution of genetics to the pathogenesis of PCOS is not due to a single gene but inheritance of gene clusters [3]. The metabolic dysfunction in PCOS patients mainly reflects molecular dysfunction of insulin signaling pathway, mainly at the level of the skeletal muscle and of the adipose tissue. These defects seem to be partly intrinsic and partly acquired because of hormonal and metabolic situation. Androgens, bioactive mediators (adipokines) and other pro-inflammatory molecules contribute to the altered action of insulin on peripheral tissues.

Insulin acts as a regulator of glucose balance by stimulating the uptake of glucose from insulin-sensitive tissues, such as adipose tissue and skeletal and cardiac muscle, and suppressing hepatic glucose production. Insulin is also able to suppress lipolysis leading to a decrease in free fatty acid levels (FFAs), which can mediate the action of insulin on the hepatic production of glucose. Insulin resistance is defined as a decreased ability of insulin to carry out these metabolic actions inherent in the uptake of glucose, the production of glucose and lipolysis, which then leads to the need for more circulating insulin to maintain the same effects. Thus insulin resistance is characterized by increased circulating levels of insulin, both basal and after loading glucose, if pancreatic function is normal [4].

2. Clinical aspects of PCOS

A biochemical and clinical hyperandrogenism of ovarian origin and to a lesser extent adrenal is evident in about 60–80% of PCOS patients, resulting in one of the main features of the syndrome [5]. Ovarian hyperandrogenism is mainly due to a defect in the intrinsic steroid synthesis in ovarian thecal cells. Extra-ovarian factors, such as high levels of LH and insulin and low levels of FSH, and intraovarian factors, such as anti-Müllerian hormone (AMH) and inhibin, may enhance the hyperandrogenism state. Also high levels of androgens are recognized as one of the possible causes of PCOS insulin resistance. An excess of androgens during intrauterine life and in the immediate postnatal period may lead to accentuate visceral adiposity and insulin resistance. Medications with anti-androgenic activity may improve insulin resistance. Androgens by acting directly on the insulin signaling system may contribute to the peripheral insulin resistance in patients with PCOS. Insulin resistance and compensatory hyperinsulinaemia are involved in all three main clinical aspects of the syndrome: hyperandrogenaemia, ovarian dysfunction and metabolic alterations [6].

The increased pulsatility of the LH leads to increased circulating LH levels that stimulate the ovarian cortex synthesis of androgens. Increased levels of LH are partly due to an altered negative feedback exerted by androgens on the hypothalamic–pituitary axis [8]. Insulin, in synergy with LH, will enhance the stimulation of androgen production by theca cells of the ovary and to a lesser extent the adrenal cortex. Insulin is also involved in the ovarian dysfunction by increasing the expression of LH receptors on the granulosa cells [9]. The first therapeutic approach in obese patients with PCOS is to achieve weight loss. In addition to an improvement of metabolic comorbidities associated with obesity, weight loss reduces hyperinsulinaemia with a consequent increase of insulin sensitivity, decreased LH and androgen levels and improvement of both menstrual cycle and fertility [10].

Patients with PCOS have an altered metabolism of inositol, and there is a connection between insulin resistance and inositol deficiency [11]. In women with PCOS, at the level of muscle tissue, the conversion of myo-Inositol into D-chiro-inositol is reduced due to a reduction in epimerasic activity. Furthermore, these patients show reduced serum D-chiro-inositol levels and an increase in urinary excretion of inositol phosphoglycan, which is inversely related to insulin sensitivity, supporting the hypothesis according to which women with PCOS present a serious alteration of the metabolism of inositols, characterized by an excess of myo-inositol and a deficiency of D-chiro-inositol and a decrease in epimerasic activity. This hypothesis has led to focus the attention on the importance of myo-inositol and D-chiro-inositol supplementation to restore normal ovarian function [12].

3. PCOS and metabolic syndrome

The identification of the different manifestations of PCOS in the various phases of the life, can, of course, help to organize individual therapeutic strategies and likely to prevent long-term metabolic consequences. Women with PCOS may have different degrees of insulin resistance (IR) that contribute to the increased risk of metabolic syndrome. The latter, defined in the past as "syndrome X" or "insulin resistance syndrome" or "plurimetabolic syndrome", is described by the association of various metabolic disorders, each of which is a known cardiovascular risk factor.

The definition of metabolic syndrome according to the National Cholesterol Education Expert Panel (NCEP) on Detection, Evaluation, and Treatment of High Blood Cholesterol in Adults (Adult Treatment Panel III—ATPIII) provides for the presence of three or more disorders between:

1. Central obesity (waist circumference ≥88 cm).

2. Impaired glucose levels (fasting blood sugar ≥110 or ≥140 mg/dl after 2 hours after oral glucose test (OGTT)).

3. Arterial hypertension (PA ≥ 130/85).

4. Hypertriglyceridaemia (≥150 mg/dl).

5. Reduced HDL cholesterol (<50 mg/dl).

These criteria are most frequently used in scientific research [13].

The presence of obesity in women with PCOS results in the worsening of the clinical presentation, both from a metabolic and reproductive point of view [14]. Obese women with PCOS present:

1. Increased prevalence of impaired fasting glucose (IFG) and type 2 diabetes mellitus.

2. Higher prevalence of hirsutism (73% of obese vs. 56% of non-obese) [15].

3. Worst lipid profile.

4. Increased risk of metabolic syndrome and, therefore, cardiovascular diseases [16].

5. Higher prevalence of oligomenorrhoea, amenorrhoea and infertility [17].

6. Lower rate of ovulation and conception in response to clomiphene citrate. and to exogenous gonadotrophins, with need for higher doses.

7. Lower percentage of pregnancies in assisted reproduction techniques (IVF, ICSI) and increased frequency of spontaneous abortions [18].

It should be noted that a greater predisposition to the metabolic syndrome has been described throughout the body mass index (BMI) range, indicating that PCOS, independently of obesity, can confer an increased risk of developing this complication, due to the intrinsic insulin resistance that characterizes it. Women with PCOS and a combination of metabolic syndrome would exhibit greater insulin resistance, higher levels of free testosterone, lower levels of SHBG and, phenotypically, greater frequency of acanthosis nigricans [16]. The prevalence of metabolic syndrome, however, would be higher in patients with high BMI than in those with normal BMI.

4. Pathophysiology

The considerable variability of the clinical presentation, together with the lack of universally accepted diagnostic criteria, has so far contributed to making it difficult to identify a clear etiology of the disease.

The three main endocrine changes of PCOS are:

1. Hyperandrogenism.

2. LH hypersecretion.

3. Hyperinsulinism.

The mechanisms by which these factors interact with each other in PCOS are extremely complex and not yet completely clarified [17].

The rapid onset of hyperandrogenism may be caused by steroid-secreting ovarian or adrenal tumors that must be ruled out in the differential diagnosis. On the contrary, the slow and progressive appearance of hyperandrogenism is often associated with medical history for a gradual increase in weight over time [19].

Several mechanisms that could determine Insulin resistance (IR) are:

- Excessive serine phosphorylation of the insulin receptor subunit.

- Mutations of the insulin receptor gene or IRS-1 (substrate of the insulin receptor, phosphorylated by its tyrosine kinase activity, Tyr-K).

- Depletion of intracellular adenosine.

- Post-receptor defect of glucose transport.

- Impaired insulin clearance in peripheral tissues.

Obesity amplifies insulin resistance and hyperinsulin state in PCOS patients, and that, therefore, obese patients are more insulin-resistant and more hyperinsulinaemic of the normal-weight counterpart. Despite the peripheral insulin resistance, ovarian tissue remains sensitive to action of insulin, probably because at this level, the transduction system involves a different second messenger, inositol phosphoglycan.

So, insulin can act directly on the cells of the ovary, activating cytochrome P450c17 and enhancing the synthesis of androgen induced by LH. The increased proactive androgenic action of insulin also manifests itself indirectly, by suppressing the hepatic synthesis of sex hormone-binding globulin (SHBG) and insulin-like grow factor-binding protein 1 (IGFBP-1), with consequent increase in the bioavailability of free testosterone of IGF-I. The latter would act by stimulating the secretion of progesterone and oestradiol and increasing the aromatase activity and production of androgens, respectively, in granulosa and thecal cells (**Figure 1**).

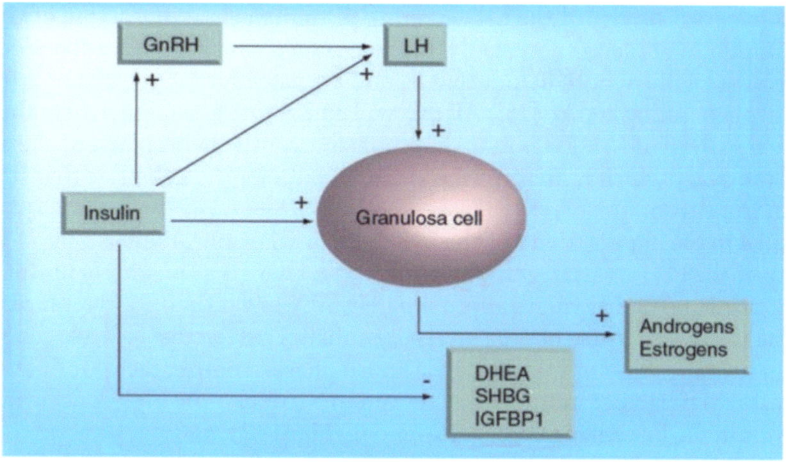

Figure 1.
Insulin actions and androgen production [7].

Insulin acts by modifying the pulsatile secretion of GnRh increasing the sensitivity of gonadotropic cells to GnRh.

An important role to the genesis of insulin resistance has been attributed to free fatty acids (FFA) [20]. The visceral adipocytes of women with PCOS have increased the lipolytic activity of abdominal fat with subsequent marked lipolytic activity that enhances the massive release of FFA in the portal blood. FFAs once they reach the liver trigger an inflammatory parenchymal state, induce a reduction in androgen clearance and inhibition of SHBG synthesis, but above all inhibit the hepatic extraction of circulating insulin. In this way FFA contribute to peripheral hyperinsulinaemia. FFA also compete with glucose as the energy substrate of skeletal muscles [21], and with this modality, they would contribute to the genesis of insulin resistance.

A contribution to hyperinsulinaemia also comes from a secretory pancreatic defect, found in some patients with PCOS even in the absence of glucose intolerance or a frank type 2 diabetes [22]. In particular, an exaggerated pancreatic secretion was demonstrated in the first phase of the response to a hypoglycaemic stimulus administered in order to test pancreatic secretory capacity. This anomaly is present in lean PCOS as well as in obese PCOS resulting in a defect independent of other confounding factors such as BMI, adipose tissue distribution, peripheral sensitivity to insulin or a family history of noninsulin-dependent diabetes mellitus (NIDDM).

From the neuroendocrine point of view, PCOS represents distinctive feature of the inappropriate secretion of gonadotrophins. There are numerous studies that demonstrate the existence of an alteration of the hypothalamic–pituitary-ovary axis which is expressed on the hormonal level in:

- An increase in the secretion of LH: in particular, an increase in the amplitude and frequency of the LH observed in basal conditions [23].

- The relative suppression of FSH suggests that partial pituitary desensitization is secondary to the increased frequency of GnRH secretion [23].

An alteration of the circadian rhythm of LH is also observed with persistence of nocturnal hyperactivity typical of adolescence. This suggests the existence of a marked hypersensitivity of the LH-secreting pituitary cells to the action of GnRH [24]. Another hypothesis suggests the presence of a partial loss of feedback control mechanisms on the hypothalamus that lead to a greater autonomy of the GnRH pulsatility generating centre [25]. All this will contribute to irregularity in the hormonal pattern of LH. LH is in turn responsible for the hyperplasia of the theca cells of the ovary which represents the anatomopathological substrate that supports hyperandrogenism.

Parallel to the hyperactivity of the LH-theca ovarian axis, there is a hypo-functionality of the FSH-ovarian granulosa axis: in fact here is a constantly uniform FSH concentration, settled at values approximately 30% lower than the reference values [26]. The relative decrease of FSH levels my enhance a defective folliculogenesis that lead to maturation of follicles at the antral phase. Another factor influencing anovulation is the hyperandrogenic state and in particular the high concentration of androgens in the follicular microenvironment (**Figure 2**).

Two other important mechanisms of action of insulin are responsible for hyperandrogenaemia:

1. The inhibition of the hepatic synthesis of SHBG (sex hormone-binding globulin), which determines a greater bioavailability of free oestrogens and androgens [27].

2. The inhibition of hepatic production of IGFBP-1 (insulin-like growth factor-binding protein-1) which increases the circulating levels of IGF-1 and its activity [28, 29]. Among the various actions, IGF-1 also appears to stimulate the activity of the enzyme 5α-reductase, responsible for converting testosterone into dihydrotestosterone, its active metabolite.

The concentration of insulin-like growth factor-binding protein-1 (IGFBP-1) is directly correlated to the degree of obesity, in fact overweight reduces its concentrations even in non-PCOS women. As a result, obesity also plays an essential role in the pathogenesis of hyperandrogenism in PCOS, as BMI is the main determinant of IGFBP-1 Levels [29].

There is evidence that a vitamin D deficiency could be involved in the genesis of insulin resistance and metabolic syndrome in PCOS and would also play a role in determining the hormonal status of PCOS patients [30, 31].

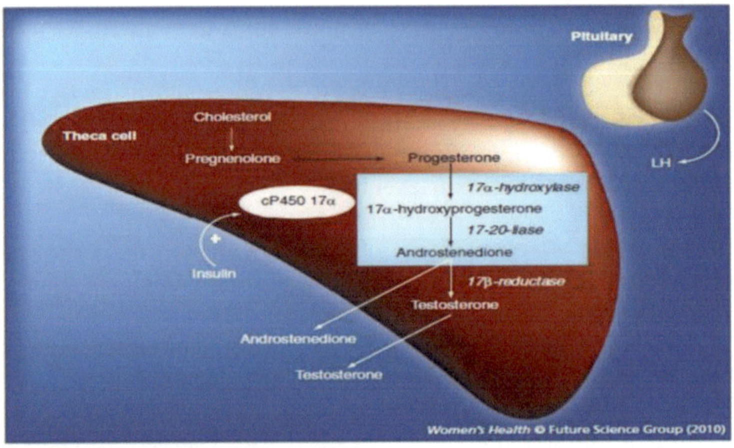

Figure 2.
Insulin action on the theca cell steroidogenesis [7].

5. Clinical evaluation: Diagnostic criteria for PCOS in adult women

The prevalence of PCOS varies according to the diagnostic criteria used which usually include extension of hirsutism, level of circulating androgens, degree of irregularity of the menstruation and ultrasound morphology of the ovary.

Patients suffering from PCOS most frequently complain of:

1. Menstrual irregularities: usually associated with anovulation which is the cause of oligomenorrhoea (less than nine menstrual cycles per year; cycles of average duration exceeding 36–40 days). Anovulation in 30% of cases is accompanied by secondary amenorrhoea (no menstrual periods for three or more consecutive months) which occurs after a period of variable oligomenorrhoea.

2. Hyperandrogenism. The most characteristic clinical presentations are hirsutism and acne. Total testosterone is the best to reflect the androgenic status as the free testosterone level may not be very accurate. Total testosterone can be measured on any day of the menstrual cycle [32]. Other laboratory investigations that can be made are:

    - Free androgen index (FAI) is the ratio between total testosterone and SHBG.
    - Androstenedione is the direct precursor of testosterone, produced by the ovaries, adrenals and peripheral tissues. In women with PCOS, androstenedione levels can be increased even when the total testosterone is normal [33].
    - DHEA-S is almost exclusively of adrenal origin and is increased in about 20–30% of PCOS patients. Hyperandrogenaemia, therefore, is predominantly of ovarian origin and supported by the increased activity of the P450c17 enzyme complex in thecal cells, which has two activities, 17α-hydroxylase, which converts progesterone to 17-OH-P, and 17–20 lyase, which transforms the latter into androstenedione (**Figure 2**). Androstenedione will then be converted into testosterone by 17β-hydroxysteroid dehydrogenase. In particular, the activity of 17α-hydroxylase is increased. Furthermore, it appears to be an adrenal contribution to hyperandrogenaemia, again due to the excessive activation of the same microsomal enzyme P450c17, predominantly in the activity of 17–20 lyase, although a hyper-responsiveness to ACTH is not to be excluded. Insulin is able to directly stimulate the enzymatic activity of P450c17, both at the adrenal and ovarian level [34]. A recent study has shown that androstenedione and total testosterone level helps to better assess the risk of developing metabolic syndrome in women with PCOS [33].

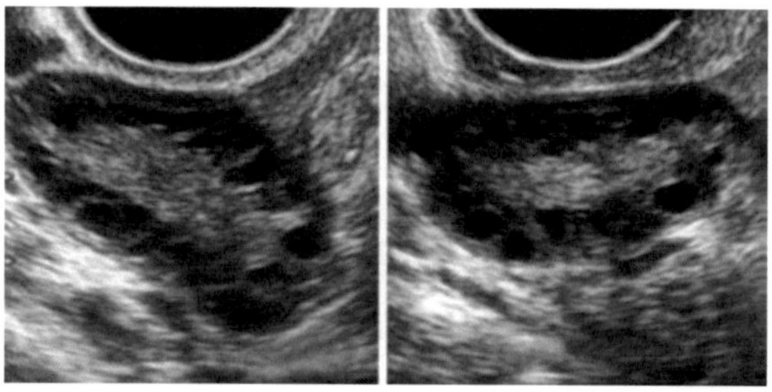

Figure 3.
Ultrasound imaging of polycystic ovaries [35].

3. Polycystic ovary morphology: according to the Rotterdam criteria, the ovaries are defined as "polycystic" at least 1 ovary showing 12 or more follicles with average diameter 2–9 mm, regardless of their disposition, and/or a total ovarian volume >10 ml^3, examined with a transvaginal probe, and the evaluation must be carried out both in longitudinal and transverse scanning plane. It is sufficient that only one ovary has these characters, if evaluated in the follicular phase and in the absence of any hormonal treatment. Peripheral distribution of the follicles and hypertrophy of the ovarian stroma may be present but are not necessary for diagnosis (**Figure 3**).

6. Therapeutic approach

Therapeutic choices will be based on the type and extent of the disorders and if there is a desire for pregnancy.

The goals of the therapeutic action are:

- Improvement in menstrual cycles
- Reduce circulating androgens and signs of hyperandrogenism
- Reduce insulin resistance and prevent metabolic complications and decrease cardiovascular risk
- Try to achieve the ideal weight
- Treatment of infertility and improving the response to ovulation induction therapies
- Endometrial protection to prevent endometrial carcinoma

The therapeutic options available for PCOS are represented by lifestyle changes and the use of oral contraceptives, androgen receptor antagonists and insulin-sensitizing drugs such as metformin and inositol-based supplements.

The first therapeutic approach in women with PCOS must be represented by lifestyle changes, by nutrition and in the presence of obesity or overweight by weight loss. In addition to an improvement in the metabolic comorbidities associated with obesity, weight loss reduces hyperinsulinaemia and increases insulin sensitivity, leading also to a decrease in LH and androgen levels.

Palomba et al. demonstrated in two cohorts of patients followed for 24 weeks, one of which was subjected to a regular exercise programme while the other to hypocaloric hyperproteic diet, in both cases there was a decrease in insulin resistance and improvement in menstrual cycles, fertility, SHBG and androgen levels [36].

Improvements of ovulation were found after weight loss in the PCOS obese patient as weight reduction could play the most significant role in restoring ovulation [37].

6.1 The use of combined oral contraceptive (COC) pill

This treatment produces regular menstrual cycles, decreases the risk of endometrial hyperplasia and improves acne and hirsutism. The treatment with COC pill represents therefore the therapy of first choice for the treatment of hyperandrogenism.

COC treatment increases the hepatic synthesis of SHBG, reducing the proportion of free and therefore metabolically active testosterone. Among the progestogens that can be used in various associations, those with anti-androgenic activity are preferred, such as cyproterone acetate (which acts by preventing the binding of androgens to their cellular receptors) and drospirenone (which is a progestin with an anti-androgenic and anti-mineralocorticoid action).

6.2 Insulin-sensitizing treatment

The rationale of the use of insulin sensitizers in PCOS derives from the fact that 45–65% of PCOS patients have insulin resistance and compensatory hyperinsulinaemia [38] which alter the steroidogenesis of the ovary and follicular maturation [39].

The classic insulin-sensitizing treatment is metformin, a biguanide traditionally used in the treatment of people with type 2 diabetes. Metformin acts by increasing the uptake and utilization of glucose at the level of skeletal muscle and adipose tissue by reducing the insulin resistance and decreasing hepatic gluconeogenesis; it is also able to reduce intestinal glucose absorption and lipolysis, causing the reduction of substrates for gluconeogenesis.

Metformin has a significant effect on the reduction in circulating androgen levels, weight loss and regularization of menstrual cycles and ovulatory cycles [40].

Metformin action on androgens and the mechanisms by which metformin acts on hyperandrogenaemia are:

- Reduced production of androgens in the ovaries [41] and adrenals [42].
- Reduced pituitary secretion of LH [43].
- Increased SHBG liver production [44].

6.3 Inositol

It exerts an important control over glucose homeostasis, and when incorporated into phosphoglycans, it functions as an intracellular mediator of the action of insulin.

Inositol improves insulin sensitivity and ovulation rate, decreasing the testosterone concentration, blood pressure and plasma triglyceride concentrations [45].

The insulin-sensitizing action of inositol is the myo-inositol and the D-chiro-inositol. The conversion of myo-inositol into D-chiro-inositol by the epimerase is dependent on insulin, so the liver and muscle (the insulin-sensitive tissues) are those in which the greatest conversion occurs. They are both chemical mediators of insulin. The activation of phospholipids containing myo-inositol by insulin causes an increase in the permeability of the cell membrane to glucose with consequent increase in its internalization and availability for use. D-chiro-inositol, on the other hand, may allow the intracellular accumulation of glucose in the form of glycogen. The result of the action of both is however the increase in insulin sensitivity with consequent reduction in the circulating levels of insulin [46].

7. Conclusion

PCOS is a widespread pathology that affects multiple aspects of the general health of women, with long-term effects that go well beyond the reproductive age.

The term "polycystic ovary syndrome" does not completely reflect the complexity of this syndrome which manifests a wide spectrum of clinical manifestations and comorbidity and important metabolic implications. PCOS patients showed an increase risk of developing type 2 diabetes mellitus, dyslipidaemia, endometrial cancer and cardiovascular diseases.

The main features of PCOS are hyperandrogenism, oligomenorrhoea and ultrasound morphology of the ovary.

PCOS is also associated with reduced fibrinolytic activity due to increased levels of inhibitor of the plasminogen activator (PAI-I), independently of body mass index, as it is also found in thin women suffering from this syndrome and appears to correlate with the risk of abortion [47].

Atypical endometrial hyperplasia, whose incidence is increased, seems to be due both to chronic exposure to high levels of oestrogens, not balanced by an adequate amount of progesterone (due to chronic anovulation).

Patients with PCOS also have reproductive alterations, evidence of insulin resistance, anxiety and depression. If pregnant, these women have a significant increase in the risk of developing gestational complications like miscarriage, gestational diabetes, pre-eclampsia and preterm birth [48].

The mechanisms that could determine insulin resistance (IR) areexcessive serine phosphorylation of the insulin receptor subunit, mutations of the insulin receptor gene, depletion of intracellular adenosine, post-receptor defect of glucose transport and impaired insulin clearance in the peripheral tissues.

The PCOS Consensus Workshop Group in Rotterdam in which the diagnostic criteria were reviewed, allowing a broader spectrum of PCOS phenotypes to be included in the diagnosis defining PCOS as the presence of at least two of the following criteria after excluding other causes of hyperandrogenism [49], is as follows:

- Oligo-anovulation
- Hyperandrogenism with clinical or biochemical signs
- Polycystic ovary appearance on ultrasound examination

The therapeutic choices will be based on the type and extent of the disorders and if there is a desire for pregnancy.

The goals of the therapeutic action are to reduce circulating androgens and signs of hyperandrogenism, reduce insulin resistance and prevent metabolic complications and decrease cardiovascular risk.

Author details

Bassim Alsadi
Rome University 'La Sapienza', Rome, Italy

*Address all correspondence to: balsadi@hotmail.com

References

[1] Sirmans SM, Pate KA. Epidemiology, diagnosis, and management of polycystic ovary syndrome. Clinical Epidemiology. 2013;**6**:1-13

[2] Jahanfar S, Seppala M, Eden JA, Nguyen TV, Warren P. A twin study of polycystic-ovary-syndrome. Fertility and Sterility. 1995;**63**(3):478-486

[3] Legro RS, Driscoll D, Strauss JF, Fox J, Dunaif A. Evidence for a genetic basis for hyperandrogenemia in polycystic ovary syndrome. Proceedings of the National Academy of Sciences of the United States of America. 1998;**95**(25):14956-14960

[4] Kahn CR. The molecular mechanism of insulin action. Annual Review of Medicine. 1985;**36**:429-451

[5] Franks S. Diagnosis of polycystic ovarian syndrome: In defense of the Rotterdam criteria. The Journal of Clinical Endocrinology and Metabolism. 1 March 2006;**91**(3):786-789

[6] Diamanti-Kandarakis E. Polycystic ovarian syndrome: Pathophysiology, molecular aspects and clinical implications. Expert Reviews in Molecular Medicine. 2008;**10**:E3

[7] Genazzani AD, Ricchieri F, Lanzoni C. Use of metformin in the treatment of polycystic ovary syndrome. Women's Health (London, England). 2010;**6**(4):577-593

[8] Jonard S, Dewailly D. The follicular excess in polycystic ovaries, due to intra-ovarian hyperandrogenism, may be the main culprit for the follicular arrest. Human Reproduction Update. 2004;**10**(2):107-117

[9] Diamanti-Kandarakis E, Argyrakopoulou G, Economou F, Kandaraki E, Koutsilieris M. Defects in insulin signaling pathways in ovarian steroidogenesis and other tissues in polycystic ovary syndrome (PCOS). The Journal of Steroid Biochemistry and Molecular Biology. 2008;**109**(3-5):242-246

[10] Jensterle MJA, Mlinar B, Marc J, Prezelj J, Pfeifer M. Impact of metformin and rosiglitazone treatment on glucose transporter 4 mRNA expression in women with polycystic ovary syndrome. European Journal of Endocrinology. 2008;**158**:793-801

[11] Baillargeon JP, Iuorno MJ, Apridonidze T, Nestler JE. Uncoupling between insulin and release of a d-chiro-inositol-containing inositolphosphoglycan mediator of insulin action in obese women with polycystic ovary syndrome. Metabolic Syndrome and Related Disorders. 2010;**8**(2):127-136

[12] Vittorio Unfer JEN, Kamenov ZA, Prapas N, Facchinetti F. Effects of inositol(s) in women with PCOS: a systematic review of randomized controlled trials. International Journal of Endocrinology. 2016;**2016**:1849162

[13] Essah PA et al. Metabolic syndrome in women with polycystic ovary syndrome. Fertility and Sterility. 2006;**86**(Suppl 1):S18-S19

[14] Salehi M et al. Pathogenesis of polycystic ovary syndrome: what is the role of obesity? Metabolism. 2004;**53**(3):358-376

[15] Kiddy DS et al. Differences in clinical and endocrine features between obese and non-obese subjects with polycystic ovary syndrome: An analysis of 263 consecutive cases. Clinical Endocrinology. 1990;**32**(2):213-220

[16] Apronidaze T et al. Prevalence and characteristics of the metabolic

syndrome in women with polycystic ovary syndrome. The Journal of Clinical Endocrinology and Metabolism. 2005;**90**(4):1929-1935

[17] Gambineri A et al. Obesity and the polycystic ovary syndrome. International Journal of Obesity and Related Metabolic Disorders. 2002;**26**(7):883-896

[18] Pasquali R et al. Obesity and the reproductive disorders in women. Human Reproduction Update. 2003;**9**(4):359-372

[19] Snyder BS. Polycystic ovary syndrome (PCOS) in the adolescent patient: Recommendations for practice. Pediatric Nursing. 2005;**31**(5):416-421

[20] Martin ML, Jensen MD. Effects of body fat distribution on regional lipolysis in obesity. The Journal of Clinical Investigation. 1991;**88**:609

[21] Randle PJ, Hales CN, Garland PB, Newsborne EA. The glucose fatty-acid cycle. Its role in insulin sensitivity and the metabolic disturbances of diabetes mellitus. Lancet. 1963;**1**:785

[22] Dunaif A, Finegood D. β-Cell dysfunction independent of obesity and glucose intolerance in the polycystic ovary syndrome. The Journal of Clinical Endocrinology and Metabolism. 1996;**81**:942

[23] Waldstreicher J, Santoro NF, Hall JE, Filicori M, Crowley WF. Hyperfunction of the hypotalamic–pituitary axis in women with polycystic ovarian disease: Indirect evidence for partial gonadotroph desensitization. The Journal of Clinical Endocrinology and Metabolism. 1 January 1988;**66**(1):165-172

[24] Rebar R, Judd HL, Yen SSC, Rakoff J, Vendenberg G, Naftolin F. Characterization of the inappropriate gonadotropin secretion in polycystic ovary syndrome. The Journal of Clinical Investigation. 1976;**57**:1320-1329

[25] Christman GM, Randolph JF, Kelch RP, Marshall JC. Reduction of gonadotropin-releasing hormone pulse frequency is associated with subsequent selective follicle stimulating hormone secretion in women with polycystic ovary syndrome. The Journal of Clinical Endocrinology and Metabolism. 1991;**72**:1278-1285

[26] Yen SSC, Vela P, Rankin J. Inappropriate secretion of follicle-stimulating hormone and luteinizing hormone in polycystic ovarian disease. The Journal of Clinical Endocrinology and Metabolism. 1970;**30**:435

[27] Bach LA. The insulin-like growth factor system: Basic and clinical aspects. Australian and New Zealand Journal of Medicine. 1999;**29**:355-361

[28] Le Roith D, McGuinness M, Shemer J, Stannard B, Lanau F, Faria TN, et al. Insulin-like, growth factors. Biological Signals. 1992;**1**(4):173-181

[29] Kelly CJ, Stenton SR, Lashen H. Insulin-like growth factor binding protein-1 in PCOS: a systematic review and meta-analysis. Human Reproduction Update. 2011;**17**(1):4-16

[30] Alvarez JA, Ashraf A. Role of vitamin D in insulin secretion and insulin sensitivity for glucose homeostasis. International Journal of Endocrinology. 2010;**2010**:351-385

[31] Ngo DT, Chan WP, Rajendran S, et al. Determinants of insulin responsiveness in young women: Impact of polycystic ovarian syndrome, nitric oxide, and vitamin D. Nitric Oxide. 2011;**25**(3):326-330

[32] Trikudanathan S. Polycystic ovarian syndrome. The Medical Clinics of North America. 2015;**99**(1):221-235

[33] O'Reilly MW, Taylor AE, Crabtree NJ, et al. Hyperandrogenemia predicts metabolic phenotype in polycystic ovary syndrome: The utility of serum androstenedione. Journal of Clinical Endocrinology & Metabolism. 2014;**99**(3):1027-1036

[34] Qin KN, Rosenfield RL. Role of cytochrome P450c17 in polycystic ovary syndrome. Molecular and Cellular Endocrinology. 1998;**145**(1-2):111-121

[35] Balen AH, Laven JSE, Tan SL, Dewailly D. Ultrasound assessment of the polycystic ovary: International consensus definition. Human Reproduction Update. 2003;**9**:505-514

[36] Palomba SGF, Falbo A, et al. Structured exercise training programme versus hypocaloric hyperproteic diet in obese polycystic ovary syndrome patients with anovulatory infertility: A 24-week pilot study. Human Reproduction. 2008;**23**(3):642-650

[37] Hoeger KM, Kochman L, Wixom N, Craig K, Miller RK, Guzick DS. A randomized, 48-week, placebo-controlled trial of intensive lifestyle modification and/or metformin therapy in overweight women with polycystic ovary syndrome: A pilot study. Fertility and Sterility. 2004;**82**(2):421-429

[38] Palomba S, Falbo A, Zullo F, Orio F Jr. Evidence-based and potential benefits of metformin in the polycystic ovary syndrome: A comprehensive review. Endocrine Reviews. 2009;**30**(1):1-50

[39] Dunaif A, Segal KR, Shelley DR, Green G, Dobrjansky A, Licholai T. Evidence for distinctive and intrinsic defects in insulin action in polycystic-ovary-syndrome. Diabetes. 1992;**41**(10):1257-1266

[40] Velazquez EM, Mendoza S, Hamer T, Sosa F, Glueck CJ. Metformin therapy in polycystic ovary syndrome reduces hyperinsulinemia, insulin resistance, hyperandrogenemia, and systolic blood pressure, while facilitating normal menses and pregnancy. Metabolism: Clinical and Experimental. 1994;**43**(5):647-654

[41] Nestler JEJD. Decreases in ovarian cytochrome P450c17 alpha activity and serum free testosterone after reduction of insulin secretion in polycystic ovary syndrome. The New England Journal of Medicine. 1996;**335**(9):617-623

[42] La Marca AMG, Paglia T, Ciotta L, Cianci A, De Leo V. Effects of metformin on adrenal steroidogenesis in women with polycystic ovary syndrome. Fertility and Sterility. 1999;**72**:985-989

[43] Coyral-Castel S, Tosca L, Ferreira G, Jeanpierre E, Rame C, Lomet D, et al. The effect of AMP-activated kinase activation on gonadotrophin-releasing hormone secretion in GT1-7 Cells and its Potential Role in Hypothalamic Regulation of the Oestrous Cyclicity in Rats. Journal of Neuroendocrinology. 2008;**20**:335-346

[44] Bailey CJ, Turner RC. Metformin. The New England Journal of Medicine. 1996;**334**:574-579

[45] Nestler JE, Jakubowicz DJ, Reamer P, et al. Ovulatory and metabolic effects of D-chiroinositol in the polycystic ovary syndrome. England Journal of Medicine. 1999;**340**:1314-1320

[46] Huang LC, Fonteles MC, Houston DB, Zhang C, Larner J. Chiroinositol deficiency and insulin resistance. III. Acute glycogenic and hypoglycemic effects of two inositol phosphoglycan insulin mediators in normal and streptozotocin-diabetic rats in vivo. Endocrinology. 1993;**132**(2):652-657

[47] Gluek CJ, Wang P, Fountaine RN. Plasminogen activator inhibitor activity:

An independent risk factor for the high miscarriage rate during pregnancy in women with polycystic ovary syndrome. Metabolism. 1999;**48**:1589-1595

[48] Boomsma CM, Eijkemans MJ, Hughes EG, Visser GH, Fauser BC, Macklon NS. A meta-analysis of pregnancy outcomes in women with poly-cystic ovary syndrome. Human Reproduction Update. 2006;**12**:673-683

[49] Roterdam ESHRE/ASRM Sponsored PCOS Consensus Workshop Group. Revised 2003 consensus on diagnostic criteria and long-term health risks related to polycystic ovary syndrome. Fertility and Sterility. 2004;**81**:19-24

Chapter 2

Clinical Impact of Insulin Resistance in Women with Polycystic Ovary Syndrome

Maria Mitkova Orbetzova

Abstract

Polycystic ovary syndrome (PCOS) is an endocrine-metabolic disorder characterized by multiple hormonal imbalances, reflecting on the clinical presentation. Among them, the insulin resistance (IR), defined as a metabolic state characterized by a decrease in cellular ability to respond to insulin signaling, is a key feature of PCOS independently of obesity. Thus, IR occurs in more than 70% of obese PCOS women and in 30–50% of lean ones. Compensatory high insulin levels are both a symptom and an underlying physiopathological driver of PCOS. Insulin appears to disrupt all components of the hypothalamic-pituitary-ovarian axis, and ovarian tissue IR results in impaired metabolic signaling but intact mitogenic and steroidogenic activity, favoring hyperandrogenemia. The latter is the main culprit of the clinical picture in PCOS. Testing for IR can be helpful to rule out other conditions that are commonly misdiagnosed as PCOS and to recommend an appropriate treatment for the different PCOS phenotypes.

Keywords: polycystic ovary syndrome, insulin resistance, obesity, adipose tissue, adipocytokines

1. Introduction

Polycystic ovary syndrome (PCOS) is emerging as one of the most common endocrine disorders, affecting about 5–14% of the women of reproductive age and a leading cause of infertility [1–3]. In recent decades, there has been a wealth of evidence that the disease is a typical example of a female sex specific metabolic syndrome (MetS) due to IR, with obesity having an additional aggravating effect [4–6]. The interest in PCOS, from its first description in 1935 by Stein and Leventhal as a combination of bilaterally enlarged polycystic ovaries with manifest hirsutism, obesity, amenorrhea/oligomenorrhea, and infertility in a group of women [7], is an ever increasing one, becoming interdisciplinary, as affected girls and young women are at increased risk of cardiovascular disease (CVD) compared to age-matched healthy women [8–10]. This opinion is based mainly on the metabolic disorders established in PCOS (**Table 1**).

PCOS is a complex disorder that results from the interaction of diverse genetic and environmental factors. Heritable factors include polycystic ovarian morphology due to functional ovarian steroidogenic defects, hyperandrogenemia, IR, and insulin secretory defects. Acquired obesity is a major postnatal unfavorable factor [11] (**Figure 1**).

Overweight/obesity (android type)
Insulin resistance/hyperinsulinemia
Impaired fasting glucose (IFG)/impaired glucose tolerance (IGT)/ Diabetes mellitus (DM) type 2
Gestational diabetes mellitus
Dyslipidemia (↓HDL-cholesterol; ↑ triglycerides)
Arterial hypertension/Arterial hypertension during pregnancy
Hypercoagulation
Hyperuricemia

Table 1.
Metabolic disorders in PCOS.

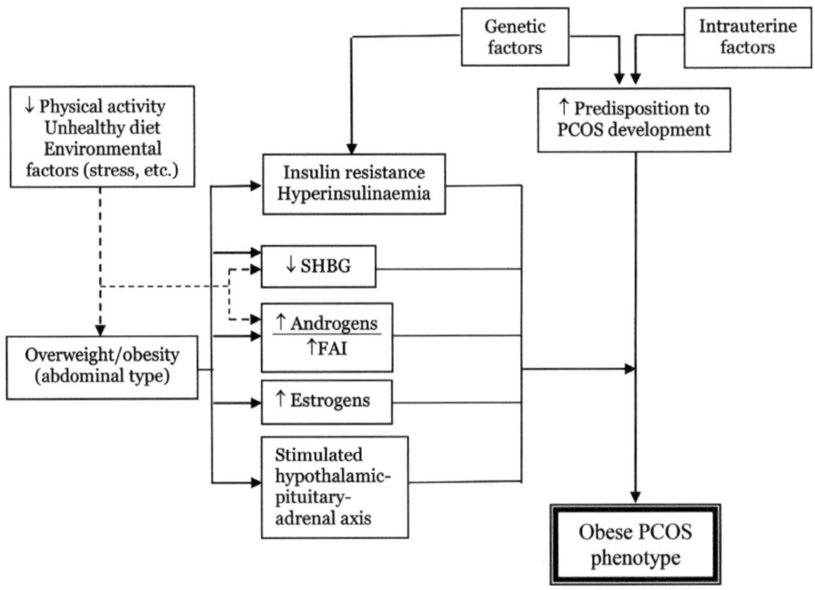

Figure 1.
Mechanisms by which obesity may determine the obese PCOS phenotype (adapted according to [11]).

The major atherogenic risk factor is IR, since excluding all other pathological abnormalities, weight included, the hyperinsulinemic women with PCOS have a 5-fold higher incidence of CVD risk factors than the normoinsulinaemic ones. But the latter, in turn, remain at a significantly higher CVD risk than their age-and BMI-matched healthy controls [12]. This fact supports the main impact of the disease itself. The role of hyperandrogenemia as an independent determinant of CVD risk in PCOS is controversial—there are studies supporting [13] and rejecting [14] the direct link; moreover, elevated androgen levels are interpreted by most authors as being secondary to an underlying IR [15–17].

Not only does the presence of hyperandrogenemia and IR/compensatory hyperinsulinemia in PCOS elucidate such important pathogenetic mechanisms of the disease, but some clinical observations show that, in fact, the late metabolic complications are more deleterious than the reproductive dysfunction itself. Moreover, recent data from a long-term prospective study indicate that hyperinsulinemia and IR tend to deepen spontaneously in PCOS women, even without worsening of the hyperandrogenism [18]. PCOS is a markedly heterogeneous disease that is why the results of numerous studies on CVD risk assessment in the PCOS women are controversial. This is due to some differences in research trial designs and the characteristics of PCOS women cohorts in terms of weight and anthropometric variables, presence or absence of IR, and other metabolic disorders [19].

2. Carbohydrate disturbances and insulin resistance in PCOS

Glucose tolerance in women with PCOS was systematically investigated for the first time by Dunaif et al. in 1987 [20]. A number of studies involving large populations of PCOS women reported incidence of *carbohydrate disturbances* higher than 40% (30–35%: IGT and 8–12%: overt DM type 2) [20, 21], which is considerably higher than the one observed in population studies of age-matched women. Overweight is a prerequisite for the development of carbohydrate disturbances, but Legro et al. [22] demonstrated that even lean PCOS women were exposed to a higher risk—31.1% had IGT and 7.5% were newly diagnosed with DM. In an Italian study, the incidence of carbohydrate disturbances was found to be lower—DM 2.5% and IGT 15.5% [23]. The Australian study of Dabadghao et al. reported incidence of overt DM 4% and IGT 15.6%, the latter correlating with age, family history, abdominal obesity, and the presence of MetS [24].

In general, the incidence of a *newly diagnosed DM* in targeted studies in PCOS women reaches 10%, the greater part of the affected women being in the third or fourth decade of life. Even the lower DM incidence in certain populations of PCOS women has proved to be significantly higher, as compared to the age-matched populations. For instance, in a study conducted at the University of Pittsburgh, DM type 2 was observed in 12.6% of PCOS women of an average age 42 years, against 1.4% observed in the corresponding healthy population [25]. In the Netherlands, DM was found in 2.3% of the normal-weight PCOS women, aged 45–54, but this incidence was four times higher, as compared to the control population [26]. Two studies of ours in Bulgaria [27, 28] found DM incidence of 1.4% in a group of 142 PCOS women and 1.1% in another group of 94 patients, which is a comparatively low figure. However, we must take into consideration that DM in PCOS women is manifested relatively later, at an age between 30 and 40, and the predominant part of our patients were of a younger age (average age 22 years). That is why special attention should be paid to the risk groups—the women with IFG and IGT (in our studies they were 4.9 and 7.4%, respectively) and especially those who are overweight or obese as well (5.8 and 6.4%, respectively) [27, 28].

The PCOS women are more predisposed to development of *gestational DM* as well [29]. On the other hand, women with gestational DM have a higher incidence of PCOS, diagnosed postpartum [30, 31], and this is associated with persistent carbohydrate disturbances occurring afterward [32], in contrast to the usual returning to the norm. A study involving diabetic PCOS women found that 55% of them had gestational DM during pregnancy [33].

Following the initial evidence of Burghen et al. concerning the presence of hyperinsulinemia in PCOS [34], many other investigators obtained similar results demonstrating that both lean and obese PCOS women are characterized by IR and hyperinsulinemia [35, 36]. It has been proved that PCOS women have a more marked IR as compared to age- and BMI-matched healthy women, the difference becoming greater with the increase in BMI [33–37]. The use of insulin sensitizers significantly improved the characteristic metabolic and endocrine features of PCOS, ovulatory function, menstrual cyclicity, and fertility [19, 38–41].

It is generally accepted that obese PCOS women are insulin-resistant. The obese PCOS women have higher insulin levels and/or more marked IR, as compared to obese controls and normal-weight PCOS women [42]. Still debatable is the issue whether IR in PCOS depends on weight and/or the android redistribution of adipose tissue, or it is intrinsic to the disease, since there is evidence in both directions [35, 43–46]. Studies differing in design have obtained similar results, showing that both obese and lean PCOS women have IR and hyperinsulinemia. Some of these differences are due mainly to nonstandardized criteria for diagnosing both PCOS and IR. Family history of DM type 2 is not always taken into account. In addition, there are certain racial and ethnic peculiarities, which become more and more distinct regarding not only the individual characteristics of PCOS, but also the insulin sensitivity and the MetS itself [47–49].

It is important to know that irrespective of the occurrence of multiple risk factors, DM develops only in the presence of *impaired β-cell function*. In addition to the reduced insulin sensitivity, secretory dysfunction in pancreatic β-cells has been found in PCOS [50, 51]. This β-cell defect—increased fasting and reduced postprandial insulin secretion—results in inability of the available insulin to compensate for the degree of resistance to its action. The reduced postprandial response to insulin in PCOS women resembles the defect typical of DM type 2 and is much more marked in those who have first-degree relatives with DM type 2. Weight reduction results in significant improvement in IR, but the β-cell defect persists [38], which presupposes that it may prove to be a primary abnormality in PCOS. This is supported by the fact that the β-cell is unable to compensate for the peripheral IR that occurs early in the course of PCOS. Thus, a reduced first phase of insulin secretion has been established in adolescent girls with PCOS, as well as reduced index of glucose disposal and increased liver glucose production [52].

As it was stated above, the PCOS women have an *increased basal insulin secretion*, although the insulin secretory response to glucose loading as a whole is inadequate, as compared to that of healthy women [43, 53]. On tissue level, IR develops in the liver, adipose tissue, and muscles of PCOS women. Hyperinsulinemia in PCOS is considered to be secondary to IR. The latter involves a new mechanism of marked defects in insulin-dependent glucose transport, with significant alterations in receptor dynamics [54]. Marked reduction in insulin sensitivity has been found in biopsy-obtained adipocytes of PCOS women, as well as a milder but also significant decrease in the maximum rate of insulin-stimulated glucose transport, secondary to the reduced expression of GLUT-4 glucose transporters [55]. Such defects are observed in DM type 2 and obesity, but in PCOS they are found even in the absence of carbohydrate disturbances, overweight, and alteration in the waist-to-hip ratio (WHR). Moreover, they do not correlate with sex hormone levels, which suggest that the impairment of insulin action is most likely primary [56].

With a view to further elucidate post-receptor defects, a reduction in insulin-dependent receptor tyrosine autophosphorylation has been found in isolated fibroblasts of about 50% of PCOS women, as well as an increase in noninsulin dependent receptor serine phosphorylation, i.e., receptor tyrosine kinase activity is inhibited. A factor extrinsic to the insulin receptor, probably serine/threonine kinase, induces serine phosphorylation of the insulin receptor, which results in signal inhibition [57, 58]. This defect leads to IR in the early stages of insulin-receptor-mediated signal transduction. This unique PCOS characteristic distinguishes it from the other clinical conditions with IR [57]. The resultant hyperinsulinemia, arising as it seems upon triggering of puberty, may involve the system of ovarian insulin-like growth factors (IGFs), influence the liver production of the IGF binding protein-1(IGFBP-1), and is probably a pathogenetic factor in the development of the disease [59].

Serine phosphorylation seems to modulate the activity of the key regulatory enzyme of androgen biosynthesis—P450c17, present in both ovarian and adrenal steroidogenic tissue. In this way, serine phosphorylation enhances enzymatic activity and increases androgen synthesis [60]. It is interesting to note that serine phosphorylation of insulin receptor substrate-1 (IRS-1) is also the mechanism of the TNF-α-mediated IR in obesity [61]. Thus, one and the same defect—serine phosphorylation—is likely to result in both IR and hyperandrogenism. This is a very tempting hypothesis explaining the syndrome pathogenesis; unfortunately, it is valid for only a part (about 50%) of the population of PCOS women.

With view to establishing a defect in insulin action after binding to the receptor, Book and Dunaif [62] investigated the metabolic and mitogenic effects of insulin and IGF-1 in a culture of skin fibroblasts from PCOS women and healthy controls. The authors found that in PCOS, a selective defect was present involving insulin metabolic but not mitogenic signaling pathways; a similar defect was found in the action of IGF-1 (this fact shows that insulin and IGF-1 stimulate glycogen synthetase by one and the same post-receptor pathways) [62]. Poretsky et al. demonstrated that the inhibition of PI-3-kinase activity did not alter insulin-induced stimulation of progesterone production in cultures of human ovarian cells [63]. On the other hand, insulin-stimulated PI-3-kinase activity in skeletal muscles of PCOS women was damaged [64]. The results suggest that the insulin regulation of steroidogenesis and glucose metabolism uses different signaling pathways, the first one remaining functionally active and probably even overstimulated by the increased insulin levels in women with IR [4] (**Figure 2**).

The hypothesis of presence of a post-receptor defect in insulin action in PCOS is consistent with the results of investigations performed on a molecular level, which have not found structural anomalies in the insulin receptor [65–67]. What exactly the defect is remains to be elucidated. An evidence provided by Ek et al. [68] suggests a selective impairment in the function of the protein kinase A-dependent hormone-sensitive enzyme lipase, which regulates the lipolytic response to catecholamines in visceral adipose tissue in lean PCOS women with mild IR. An abnormal post-receptor sensitivity to catecholamines has been observed while the antilipolytic sensitivity to insulin is preserved [68]. This anomaly differs from the impaired

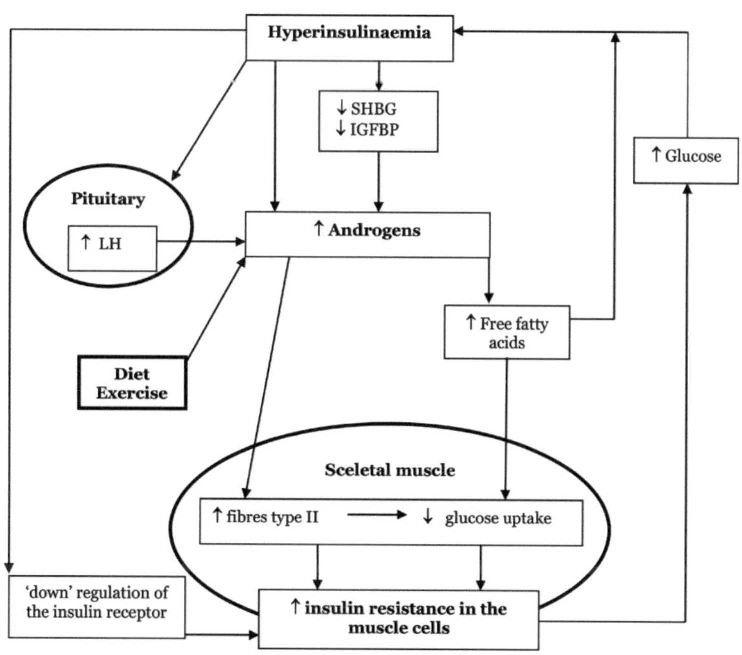

Figure 2.
Role of insulin in the pathogenesis of PCOS.

balance occurring in the MetS between the lipolytic β_3- and the antilipolytic α_2-adrenoreceptors [69]. It is still unclear whether this unique defect found in PCOS is primary or secondary to other factors, such as increased serum androgen levels.

Thus, the logical question arises—if IR and hyperinsulinemia play a major pathogenetic role in PCOS, why all women with hyperinsulinemia (e.g., with DM type 2) are not hyperandrogenic as well? IR and reproductive disturbances are probably indicative of single genetic defects and IR unmasks the syndrome in genetically predisposed individuals. Because of the fact that PCOS-related IR is a selective one and involves the metabolic but not the mitogenic and signaling pathways, we can explain the paradox of a persistent biological insulin action on reproductive processes on the background of systemic IR [70]. In general, studies have shown that predominantly PCOS women with both hyperandrogenism and chronic anovulation seem to be insulin-resistant. Women with only hyperandrogenism or a morphological finding of polycystic ovaries who have normal ovulation are less likely to develop IR [20, 71].

To sum up, *insulin and LH act synergetically on the theca-cells of the polycystic ovary* (hyperplasia of these cells is usually present) and activate *P450c17α1*; thus, enhancing the biosynthesis of ovarian androgens and testosterone [72–75]. A further adverse action of hyperinsulinemia on the ovaries of PCOS women includes arresting the development of the ovarian follicle up to 5–10 mm in size and preventing ovulation [71, 75]. Outside the ovary, insulin can act directly as a co-gonadotropin enhancing LH activity by stimulating the ovarian receptors for insulin and IGF, or indirectly by increasing the amplitude of LH serum pulses, enhancing the sensitivity to GnRH stimulation (**Figure 3**).

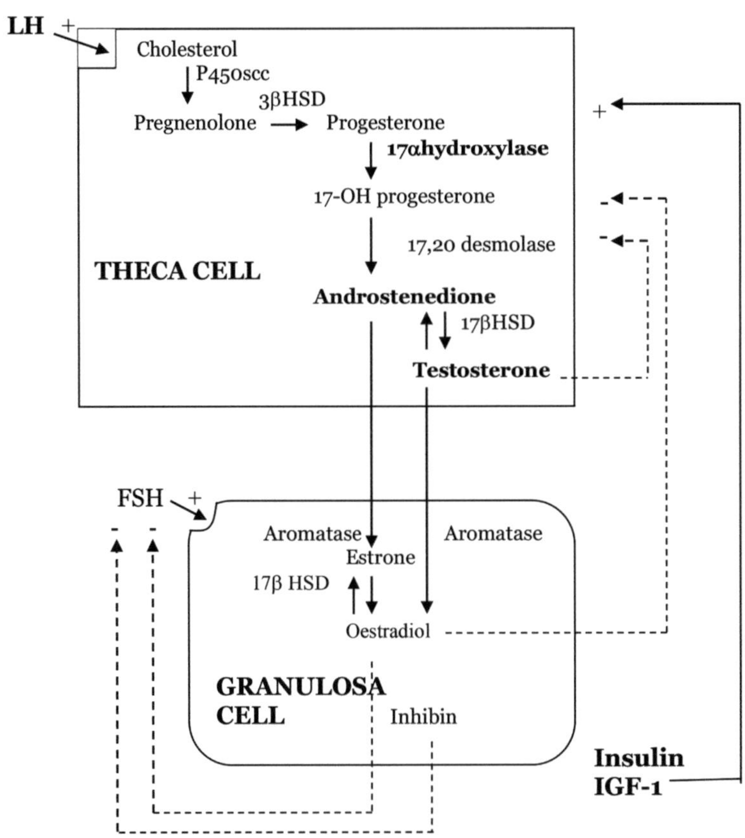

Figure 3.
Schematic representation of the factors regulating ovarian steroidogenesis.

The possible mechanism of insulin-induced enhanced ovarian steroidogenesis is supported by the higher incidence of PCOS in women with DM type 1—the ovaries of the affected women are exposed to hyperinsulinemia resulting from the availability of exogenously administered insulin in the systemic circulation [76].

In approximately 40% of the women diagnosed with PCOS in conformity with the NIH (National Institute of Health) criteria, an IGT or DM type 2 developed as sequelae of IR in the fourth decade of life, the age and weight gain having an unfavorable effect on glycemic control [27, 77–80]. In addition, a study based on the Rotterdam diagnostic criteria, 2003 reported IR in 71.54% of the studied PCOS women [81].

The incidence of IR, however, differed considerably among the various phenotypes—80.4% in the "classical" one (phenotypes A and B), 65% in the women with normal ovulation (phenotype C) and 38.1% in the group with normoandrogenemia (phenotype D). The classical phenotype and to a lesser degree the phenotype without ovulatory dysfunction were independently associated with IR, whereas in the normoandrogenic phenotype no IR was found [81]. This was confirmed by another study, showing that the number of women with PCOS and a HOMA-index >3.8 is considerably higher in the hyperandrogenic phenotypes, as compared to the normoandrogenic one [82]. That is why the nature and course of carbohydrate disturbances in women with different phenotypic presentations of PCOS require

Confirmed	Possible
Age	Chronic anovulation
Obesity	Hyperandrogenemia
Abdominal deposition of adipose tissue	Dyslipidemia (hypertriglyceridemia)
Insulin resistance	Ethnicity (certain risk populations)
β-cell dysfunction	
Family history of DM type 2	

Table 2.
Risk factors for developing carbohydrate disturbances in PCOS.

Euglycemic insulin clamp technique
Minimal model—multiple determination from i.v. GTT
Sensitivity insulin infusion tests • insulin tolerance test • insulin suppression test
Insulin parameters in oral glucose tolerance test (oGTT) • sum of insulin values • area under the insulin curve • maximal insulin/peak of insulin
Baseline insulin and derivative indexes, according to baseline blood sugar • glucose-to-insulin ratio, • HOMA-index (Homeostasis Model Assessment): fasting insulin (μIU/ml) × fasting blood sugar (mmol/l) / 22.5 • QUICKI (Quantitative Insulin Sensitivity Check Index): *1/(log (fasting insulin μU/mL) + log (fasting blood sugar mg/dL))*

Table 3.
Methods for evaluation of insulin sensitivity.

establishing a precise and timely diagnosis, as well as proper behavior by changing one's lifestyle and dietary regimen, weight reduction whenever needed, with view to reducing the risk of developing DM and/or its complications.

The risk factors for developing carbohydrate disturbances in PCOS are presented in **Table 2**.

Having in mind the incidence of carbohydrate disturbances in the general population of women aged 20–44 (7.8% for IGT and 1.0% for newly diagnosed DM type 2) and the average prevalence of PCOS (about 5%), it can be extrapolated that PCOS-associated IR contributes approximately to 20% of IGT and 40% of DM type 2 in women of reproductive age, which gives prominence to the social importance of this syndrome. In the light of this evidence in 2006, the American Association of Clinical Endocrinologists (AACE) [83] recommended screening for presence of DM in all PCOS women after the age of 30, irrespective of weight—normal or overweight. Under certain risk circumstances, screening has been recommended before that age as well [83]. Considering the fact that DM type 2 can develop with age progression, the women who have had initially a negative result should be followed-up periodically.

The methods for evaluation of insulin sensitivity are presented in **Table 3**.

In the routine clinical practice a measurement of basal and during oGTT glucose and insulin levels is most frequently used.

3. Obesity and insulin resistance in PCOS

The association between PCOS and obesity is complex. In the USA, it was reported that obesity affects from 30 to 75% of PCOS women [41, 84], which is higher than the percentage found in Europe [85, 86]. In a systematic review and meta-analysis of the literature, Lim et al. concluded that in PCOS women, as compared to the age-matched controls, a higher incidence of overweight and obesity was found [87]. In addition, the carriers of the syndrome of the Caucasian origin were found to be more overweight than their counterparts from the Asian origin [87]. These results are compromised to a certain extent by the fact that in most of the published studies, the patients have been selected from clinical practices on the basis of a subjective evaluation and local diagnostic methods. In general, overweight women are more often referred to a specialist for searching PCOS. However, in independent population samples, the incidence of obesity in PCOS does not seem as high as the one found in clinically targeted populations [27, 88]. Furthermore, PCOS incidence, based on the diagnostic criteria of NIH, is relatively stable throughout the world, irrespectively of the variable incidence of obesity in different populations [89].

In one of our studies, we found obesity in 51% and overweight of 22% in an unselected Bulgarian population of 142 women with PCOS [27]. Obesity incidence in our patients was higher than 38% found in women with PCOS from the island of Lesbos, Greece [90], and closer to the one found in England, where around 60% of the studied PCOS women were obese [71]. According to many studies including ours, PCOS women have higher ratio of central to peripheral redistribution of adipose tissue in comparison to controls [27, 91–94]. Obesity, of visceral type mainly, plays a key role in developing and maintaining the syndrome [95, 96] and influences significantly its severity as well as metabolic and CVD risk, since it is a well-known risk factor for IGT and DM type 2, IR and dyslipidemia [91, 97, 98]. In this respect, insulin sensitizers may exert complex positive effects on both metabolic consequences and clinical manifestations of hyperandrogenism in women with PCOS [19, 47, 48, 83, 91] (**Figure 4**).

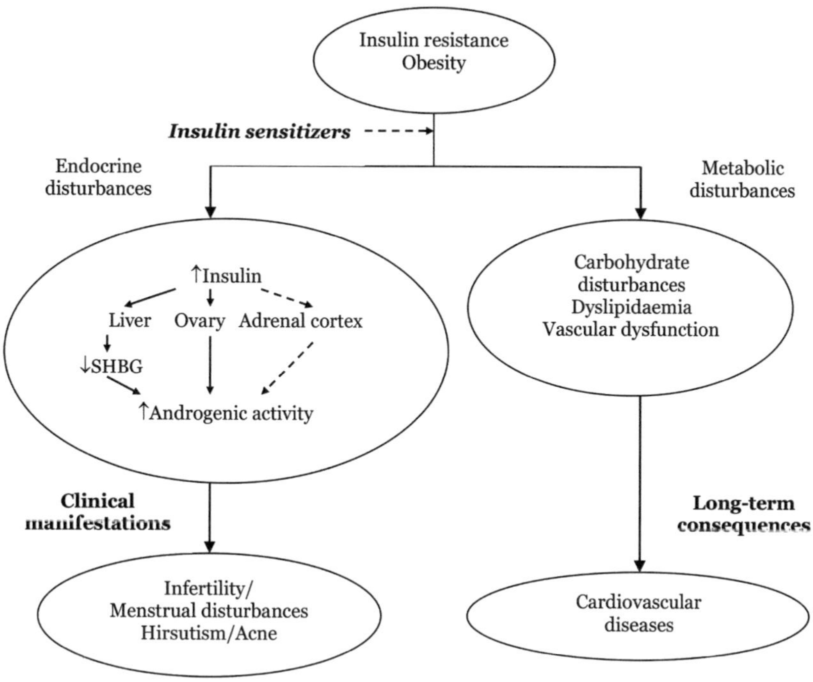

Figure 4.
Role of insulin sensitizers in the treatment of PCOS.

Obesity may promote the onset and exacerbate other long-term sequalae of PCOS, including metabolic disorders, the occurrence of some types of carcinoma, potentiated by chronic unopposed estrogen secretion, and leads to further impairing of the quality of life (QOL), low self-esteem, and worsened social adaptation, which may even potentiate occurrence of mental disorders. Obese PCOS women have a more severe clinical picture with higher incidence of IR, hyperinsulinemia, carbohydrate and lipid disturbances, and hyperandrogenism. Many studies, including ours, have shown that overweight PCOS women possess a higher degree of IR in comparison to the lean ones [27, 91–94].

Data exist that even normal-weight carriers of the syndrome show unfavorable abdominal redistribution of adipose tissue and IR [99]. In a study of young normal-weight PCOS women (mean age 15.9 ± 1.8 years, mean BMI 22.7 ± 2.3 kg/m^2) Cree-Green et al. found reduced insulin sensitivity and mitochondrial dysfunction in the muscles, relative postprandial hyperinsulinemia, abnormal glucose disposal, and increased hepatic fat in comparison to healthy controls [100].

PCOS women frequently have decreased *sex hormone-binding globulin* (*SHBG*) levels, which may decrease further with obesity development [101]. In turn, *SHBG* was found to correlate positively with HDL-cholesterol and physical activity and negatively with obesity, central distribution of adipose tissue, triglycerides, IR parameters, and presence of DM type 2 [102].

In conclusion, the concomitant obesity, especially of an android type, is associated with an increase in the long-term metabolic risk in women with PCOS.

4. Visceral adipose tissue, adipocytokines, and insulin resistance in PCOS

In the last decades, visceral adipose tissue is perceived as a source of biologically active substances—adipocytokines [103]. Commonly, PCOS women have increased amount of visceral adipose tissue and associated metabolic disorders. The influence of adipose tissue hormones on IR processes, carbohydrate, lipid, and atherogenic disorders in PCOS women is a subject of increased research interest [104].

4.1 Leptin

Leptin is known to act as a chief "adipostat"—it suppresses the intake of food and water and leads to activation of catabolic metabolic pathways related to an increased production of energy. It improves the peripheral (liver and musculoskeletal) insulin sensitivity and affects β-cell function. It has been found that there is a positive correlation between plasma leptin levels and the amount of adipose tissue in the body. Leptin levels decrease rapidly during fasting and increase after food intake. Leptin is important not only for energy balance regulation and food intake but it also performs a function of metabolic and neuroendocrine hormone; participates in glucose metabolism, reproductive processes, interacts with the *hypothalamic-pituitary*-adrenal axis; influences thyroid hormone and growth hormone secretion; and even interferes with hematopoiesis and the immune system function. There are data for a *strong association of circulating leptin and immunoreactive insulin (IRI) values and fasting plasma glucose, HOMA index, dyslipidemia, arterial hypertension that is independent or only partially dependent on obesity* [103, 104].

A close relationship between IR and hyperleptinemia in PCOS women was found irrespective of their weight [105, 106] but the results are mostly controversial due to the differences in the studies designs and the lack of data on the independent effect of obesity, as well as the presence of various phenotype expressions of PCOS. In one of our studies [107], we found higher leptin levels with borderline significance in PCOS women in comparison to age-, weight-, waist circumference-, and WHR-matched healthy controls. Significant correlation of leptin was found with BMI, waist circumference, WHR, percentage of adipose tissue, as well as with basal insulin and HOMA-index in the PCOS group [107]. These findings were confirmed and complemented by our more recent studies of women with IR syndromes, including PCOS [108, 109]. Thus, leptin exhibited significantly positive correlation with BMI, WHR, percentage of adipose tissue, basal glucose and insulin, HOMA-index, total cholesterol, triglycerides, plasma atherogenic index, Castelli I, and Castelli II indexes. A significant negative correlation was found of leptin with Matsuda index, QUICKI-index, and adiponectin [108, 109].

Mohiti-Ardekani et al. [110] also found a positive correlation between free and total leptin levels and HOMA-index in PCOS women ($r = 0.78$, $P < 0.001$; $r = 0.84$, $P = 0.003$, respectively), as well as in healthy controls ($r = 0.86$, $P < 0.001$; $r = 0.69$, $P < 0.001$, respectively). Similar results were reported by authors from Australia [111], Brazil [112], Canada [113], Finland [114], Italy [115], Sweden [116], Turkey [117] and the USA [118, 119]. In a more recent study of PCOS women (mean age 34.30 ± 2.08 years, mean BMI 34.84 ± 4.77 kg/m^2) and normally ovulating controls with comparable BMI (mean age 28.10 ± 4.61 years, mean BMI 33.59 ± 1.23 kg/m^2) Nomair et al. [120] found higher leptin concentrations in PCOS women in comparison to controls ($P = 0.005$), significant differences being found in intergroup comparative analysis between the insulin-resistant and non-insulin-resistant PCOS women as well ($P = 0.044$). In women with PCOS a positive correlation between leptin and BMI ($P = 0.049$) was found. Authors also consider BMI and IR the two chief factors associated with leptin levels [120].

Our results, as well as those from the above-mentioned studies, are indisputable proof for the role of leptin in the pathogenesis of IR in PCOS.

4.2 Adiponectin

Adiponectin is a model of an anti-inflammatory adipocytokine. A negative correlation was found between its serum levels and the degree of obesity, IR, IGT, dyslipidemia, and atherosclerosis [121–123]. The increased amount of visceral adipose tissue results in hypoadiponectinemia due to reduced expression of adiponectin genes. This leads to suppression of the insulin activity in the liver, muscles, and other peripheral tissues. Conversely, the high adiponectin levels are an independent factor for an increased insulin sensitivity and reduced risk for DM type 2. On the basis of the effects on insulin sensitivity and its anti-inflammatory properties, adiponectin is perceived as an antiatherogenic factor. The decreased adiponectin is also combined with increased production of pro-inflammatory proteins IL-6, C-reactive protein (CRP). A positive correlation between the reduced levels of the hormone and the development of ischemic heart disease has been registered [124]. It was established that adiponectin production is suppressed in conditions of IR—DM type 2 and obesity [125]. Low adiponectin levels in obesity are probably due to the process of "down"-regulation mediated by the increased amount of adipose tissue. In a study of a large population in Japan [126] and American Pima Indians [127], adiponectin levels were found to be in negative correlation with the indexes of IR even if the factors age and BMI were excluded.

Initial studies of the levels of this antiatherogenic adipocytokine in women with PCOS were conducted by Orio et al. [128] and Panidis et al. [129]. Orio et al. [128] determined serum adiponectin levels in 60 PCOS women (30 normal-weight and 30 overweight) and in 60 age- and BMI-matched healthy women. Adiponectin levels were significantly lower in obese women in comparison to normal-weight women in the PCOS group, as well as in the control group. A significant difference in adiponectin levels between PCOS women and healthy women was not found, its levels in both groups correlated negatively with BMI and HOMA-index. The authors concluded that adiponectin concentrations vary depending on the quantity of the adipose tissue and that insulin sensitivity does not play a key role in controlling adiponectin levels in PCOS women [128]. Although in other IR conditions adiponectin was found to be decreased, both cited studies reported that in normal-weight PCOS women with IR and hyperinsulinemia its levels did not differ from those in the controls [128, 129].

However, in PCOS women with severe IR, Sepilan et al. found that it was the insulin sensitivity but not the weight that was the chief determinant for adiponectin levels [130]. This fact was confirmed by one of our more recent studies [131], which revealed higher adiponectin levels in non-insulin resistant PCOS women in comparison to insulin resistant ones. In addition, insulin levels and HOMA-index proved to be higher in the group of obese PCOS women in comparison to BMI-matched controls while adiponectin levels were similar in both obese groups. On the other hand, adiponectin concentrations were significantly higher in PCOS women with normal BMI in comparison to those with obesity. In PCOS women a negative correlation between adiponectin and body weight, BMI, waist circumference, hip circumference, WHR, blood glucose at 60 and 120 min, IRI at 0, 60, and 120 min of oGTT, HOMA-index, triglycerides, triglycerides/HDL-cholesterol ratio, plasma atherogenic index, and leptin was found. We observed also a positive correlation of adiponectin with Matsuda and QUICKI indexes [109, 131]. Most probably the relation between adiponectin and IR is confined to the ability of this adipokine to stimulate glucose utilization and to reduce glucose production by the liver [71, 114]. The established significant correlation of adiponectin and androstenedione in PCOS which presupposes some interrelation between this hormone and ovarian steroidogenesis is very interesting and needs further elucidation [11, 131].

It is believed that the *leptin/adiponectin ratio (L/A)* correlates better with the degree of IR in comparison to leptin and adiponectin values taken separately. L/A is a powerful independent predictor of CVD, its values being strongly associated with the intima-media thickness and correlating positively with a number of other anthropometric, metabolic and clinical parameters [132]. In our studies we found significantly higher L/A values in PCOS women with IR in comparison to those without IR [109, 131]. This is yet another proof that insulin resistant PCOS women are with a higher CVD risk.

4.3 Resistin

Resistin, described for the first time in 2001, is a protein rich in cystein, secreted by adipocytes, and it is suspected to carry out the relationship between obesity and DM. Due to its association with obesity, inflammatory process and IR, resistin is thought to be a potential biomarker for the MetS. Thus, the higher resistin levels found in patients with overt MetS in comparison to clinically healthy individuals support this theory [133]. However, data concerning the presence of significant dependencies between resistin levels and parameters of weight and insulin sensitivity in basal conditions and following weight reduction are controversial. Some authors found significantly higher resistin levels in obese individuals in comparison to individuals with normal weight [134], while others, including us [135], did not find significant differences [136, 137].

There is controversial data in studies among PCOS women concerning resistin levels in terms of a lack of association with the syndrome [138, 139], or an increase in PCOS [140]. Thus, Panidis et al. [139] did not confirm an active role of resistin in the pathogenesis of PCOS. The authors compared anovulatory PCOS women (obese and non-obese) and healthy controls with normal weight. Resistin was significantly higher only in the obese PCOS women in comparison to the other two groups irrespectively of the differences in insulin levels and the glucose/insulin ratio. Resistin did not correlate with any hormonal or metabolite index in our Bulgarian population of PCOS women with overweight [135]. Pangaribuan et al. [141] also did not find significant difference in serum resistin levels between PCOS women and controls. Meanwhile, the authors did not find significant correlation between resistin, BMI and HOMA-index [141]. Similar serum resistin levels in normal-weight women with or without PCOS were found by Seow et al. [142]. But resistin iRNA expression in adipocytes was twice as high in PCOS women. Probably, the overexpression of the resistin gene plays a role as a local factor [142].

Olszanecka-Glinianowicz et al. [143] studied the association of adiponectin and resistin with the process of IR in PCOS women and controls. All study participants were divided into two subgroups—obese and normal-weight. Comparable serum resistin concentrations between the two subgroups of PCOS women and controls were observed. No correlations between the adipokines, HOMA-index and androgen levels were found [143]. Lewandowski et al. published similar data [144]. The authors did not find a correlation between adiponectin and resistin with the parameters of IR (basal IRI, HOMA-index, QUICKI) [144]. Yilmaz et al. obtained different results—higher resistin in PCOS women in comparison to controls, however, they observed that resistin levels remained independent of the degree of IR and BMI [145] which supports the data of some of the above-mentioned studies.

The results from our studies in adipocytokines in PCOS [47, 48, 104, 107–109, 146] showed similar resistin levels in PCOS women and metabolically healthy obese women, higher resistin levels in insulin-resistant PCOS women in comparison to non-insulin resistant ones, lack of significant difference among the different subgroups of PCOS women, divided according to BMI. Resistin correlated positively with IRI at 0 and 120 min during oGTT, HOMA-index and negatively with Matsuda and QUICKI indexes [109, 146]. Wang et al. [147] registered significantly higher resistin levels in PCOS women (obese and normal-weight) in comparison to clinically healthy women. In similarity with our data, the authors reported a positive correlation of resistin with HOMA-index and a negative one with adiponectin [147]. Resistin in our study showed a positive correlation with IL-6 [109, 146]. Our data is peculiar in this aspect since it is considered that IL-6 is the main adipocytokine which regulates resistin levels. An *in-vitro* study showed that IL-6 production, as well as the one of other cytokines (IL-1 and TNFα), increased resistin expression in mononuclear cells [148].

A number of studies on the relation of resistin with obesity, IR, MetS, CVD risk in different age populations have been conducted so far, which, though being controversial in some respects, lead to further clarification of the role of resistin in the processes of atherogenesis [149, 150]. It was found that with the increase in the number of MetS components, serum levels of resistin and other pro-inflammatory markers increase as well [150]. These and a number of other results fully support the hypothesis on the relation between circulating resistin levels and the degree of IR. Having in mind that PCOS is considered a prototype of female specific MetS in young age populations, the role of resistin has to be clarified.

4.4 Visfatin

Visfatin—a protein derived from adipose tissue that is considered to have anti-diabetic properties. Visfatin is isolated in the form of a cytokine which stimulates β-cell precursor maturation, therefore it was called *pre-β cell colony-enhancing factor (PBEF)* [151]. Visfatin stimulates glucose utilization from the adipocytes and myocytes and suppresses glucose release from liver cells, exhibiting the ability to bind to the insulin receptor and to activate it through inducing tyrosine phosphorylation. Acting as an insulin mimetic, visfatin can partially reduce IR, although it is found in much lower concentration in the circulation that insulin [152]. Visfatin participates in the process of adipocytes formation. A positive correlation between visfatin and the presence of obesity, increased visceral tissue, DM type 2 was found, and it was also elevated in patients with MetS [109, 131]. Taking in consideration these findings, the research interest in the changes in visfatin levels in PCOS is completely justified.

A meta-analysis [153] encompassing a study among 1341 women (695 with PCOS and 646 controls) showed higher visfatin levels in PCOS women without a significant correlation between it and BMI, HOMA-index, and testosterone. The authors concluded that high circulating visfatin can be perceived as a specific characteristic of PCOS, which even presupposes a role for this adipokine as a potential diagnostic biomarker for PCOS [153]. Kowalska et al. [154] found higher visfatin levels and a reduced insulin sensitivity in both normal-weight and obese PCOS women in comparison to healthy controls. Visfatin correlated negatively with parameters of IR, this correlation being well-expressed in normal-weight PCOS women, but missing in obese ones. It must be noted that in some circumstances visfatin does not succeed in exhibiting its beneficial effects on carbohydrate metabolism [154]. A hypothesis that the increase in serum visfatin levels is a secondary process aiming to prevent IR exists. On the other hand, insulin possesses the property to inhibit visfatin expression from the adipocytes so that the observed interrelationship could be explained as an inability of insulin to inhibit visfatin production in an already developed insensitivity to its action [155]. In this context, in the study of Kowalska et al. a positive correlation of visfatin with total testosterone and free androgen index (FAI) in the lean PCOS women was established [154]. The study of Tan et al. [156] also confirmed higher visfatin levels in PCOS women in comparison to age- and weight-matched healthy women. The researchers found a stimulated process of expression of visfatin mRNA and of the protein precursor of visfatin both in subcutaneous and visceral adipose tissue in PCOS women. Plasma visfatin levels were in a positive correlation with basal IRI ($P < 0.01$), HOMA-index ($P < 0.01$), testosterone ($P = 0.03$), and estradiol ($P = 0.046$). After performing a multiple regression analysis, the researchers found that the HOMA-index was the only predictive factor for visfatin levels. In contrast to plasma visfatin levels, the expressed visfatin mRNA in subcutaneous and visceral adipose tissue correlated positively with BMI and WHR [156].

In our Bulgarian studies [109, 131], we found higher serum visfatin levels in insulin-resistant PCOS women in comparison to non-insulin resistant ones. Visfatin levels in the PCOS women with obesity/overweight and in the BMI-matched metabolically healthy controls did not differ significantly. In our PCOS women, a negative correlation of visfatin with HDL-cholesterol and Matsuda index was found as well as a positive one with diastolic arterial pressure [109, 131]. In similarity to our results, Kowalska et al. reported a negative correlation between visfatin and HDL-cholesterol ($r = -0.27$, $P = 0.004$) [154]. Such negative correlation ($r = -0.349$, $P = 0.013$) was confirmed also by El-Said et al. [157] in insulin resistant PCOS women. In addition, the authors reported a positive correlation of visfatin with BMI, waist circumference, HOMA-index, FAI and a negative one with LH, total testosterone and sex hormone-binding globulin (SHBG). In this study, as well, visfatin was significantly higher in the PCOS women in comparison to the healthy women (72.94 ± 33.3 *vs* 54.69 ± 31.5 ng/mL, $P = 0.039$) [157]. In contrast to our results and the ones mentioned so far, Gen et al. reported a positive correlation between visfatin and HDL-cholesterol in normal-weight PCOS women [158].

It appears that there is controversy with respect to the relation of visfatin with insulin sensitivity indexes in women with IR and namely with PCOS and MetS. The main action of visfatin is intended at prevention of IR development as it was already pointed out, and this can explain its increase in PCOS women. The negative correlation of visfatin with IRI and HOMA-index and respectively the positive one with atherogenic indexes QUICKI and Matsuda in women with overt MetS registered in our studies is in support of this suggestion. Visfatin secretion control is a subject of increased research interest that arises much debate. Up till now, the conducted clinical studies comprising insulin resistant individuals with obesity and MetS, exhibit controversial results. The changes in this adipocytokine in PCOS women with different phenotypes are still to be clarified in targeted studies.

4.5 Tumor necrosis factor α (TNF-α) and Interleukin-6 (IL-6)

Adipose tissue is an important source of factors of low-grade inflammation not only due to the production of various cytokines by the adipocytes themselves, but also because of tissue infiltration with pro-inflammatory macrophages. The adipose tissue macrophages are responsible for the production of almost the entire amount of *TNF-α* and a significant portion of *IL-6* [159].

TNF-α is a cytokine, which interferes with the regulation of the amount of adipose tissue (inhibits the conversion of young immature fat cells into mature ones), the insulin action (disrupts the insulin receptor signal in peripheral cells) that causes post-receptor defect with subsequent development of IR [160]. The data regarding its relationship with IR are not consistent—some authors do not find any [161], but according to others insulin sensitivity is changing in parallel with the change in this cytokine levels [162, 163]. We also did not find a significant correlation of TNF-α and some parameters of IR in patients with various obesity morphotypes [135]. Basically, in our study, TNF-α levels were very similar in normal-weight women and in obese women, which corresponds to the data of Pincelli et al. [164].

It seems that the TNF-α levels, which we measure in the circulation, cannot reflect the degree of IR in obesity. It should be taken into account that this cytokine can have predominantly autocrine or paracrine action and can induce IR at a tissue level, since its concentrations *in situ*, at the level of adipose tissue, are much higher in comparison to the circulatory ones [165].

Elevated levels of TNF-α have been observed in PCOS women, which correlated positively with BMI and negatively with insulin sensitivity [166]. Gonzalez et al. [167] found elevated levels of TNF-α in normal-weight PCOS women as compared to controls. However, in all obese women in this study, despite the absence/presence of PCOS, TNF-α levels were similar. Direct correlation of TNF-α was detected with BMI, but with insulin such a correlation was found only in the healthy women. Apparently, factors other than obesity were the cause of TNF-α increase in normal-weight PCOS women. On the other hand, this cytokine did not correlate with testosterone, LH, and DHEA-S in the PCOS women [167].

We found significantly higher TNF-α concentrations in PCOS women compared to BMI-matched controls [109, 131]. In our studies, we did not establish a significant difference when comparing serum levels of TNF-α between insulin-resistant and non-insulin-resistant PCOS women. Higher levels of TNF-α were registered in obese PCOS women as compared to overweight PCOS women, but not to normal weight PCOS women. No correlations between TNF-α and the parameters of IR were established in the PCOS women [109, 131]. Contrary to our results are those of Soares et al., who did not detect a significant difference in the TNF-α levels between PCOS women and BMI-matched controls [168].

Data are controversial regarding the role of *IL-6* in the development of IR. In general, it is considered that circulating levels of IL-6 are elevated in patients with obesity and IR. It is assumed, that persistent high levels of IL-6 in chronic inflammatory conditions (obesity and DM type 2) can cause disturbances in insulin sensitivity, while only periodically elevated IL-6 levels are associated with normal carbohydrate homeostasis [162, 169]. Lin et al. suggested that IL-6 may serve as an early chronic low-grade-inflammation marker in PCOS [170]. This hypothesis, also described by other authors [171, 172], launches the idea of an association of PCOS with increased CVD risk, and the strategies affecting the chronic low-grade inflammatory conditions, can be useful for coping with PCOS and related metabolic and atherogenic disorders [173].

Mohlig et al. [174] studied IL-6 and CRP in PCOS women and in age-matched controls, analyzing the influence of C-174G-IL-6 gene polymorphism on the IL-6 and androgens levels, and on the degree of obesity. The authors did not find elevated CRP and IL-6 levels in PCOS women (both lean and obese) compared to the controls. In PCOS women the anthropometric variables (BMI, WHR, amount of adipose tissue) and the parameters of IR, but not the markers of hyperandrogenic condition, showed significant correlation with IL-6 and CRP. In addition, a 6-month metformin treatment resulted in a significant decrease in the body weight, the amount of adipose tissue and total testosterone levels, but did not affect the levels of IL-6 and CRP. Using multivariate linear regression analysis, it was established that in PCOS women BMI but not HOMA-index constituted a dominant factor explaining 18% and 24% of the variations in IL-6 and CRP levels, respectively [174].

This fact was also confirmed by another study conducted in pre-menopausal women [175]. In the study of Mohlig et al. [174], no link between the C-genotype and the IL-6 and BMI levels was found. However, the heterogeneous GC genotype was associated with lower levels of androstenedione [174]. The C-174G polymorphisms of the IL-6 gene promoter could be expected to modify its activity in certain *in vitro* conditions [176]. In some studies, C-174G polymorphism was associated with higher levels of IL-6, with more pronounced IR, with a higher degree of obesity and with hyperandrogenism [177, 178].

Our studies [107–109, 131] showed similar levels of IL-6 between the groups of PCOS women—insulin-resistant *vs* non-insulin-resistant; normal weight *vs* overweight and obese. We did not establish a significant difference in IL-6 between PCOS women and controls. Our data are in conformity with those of Villuendas et al. in women with ovarian hyperandrogenism [179], but are in confliction with the results of another study of Kelly et al. in PCOS women [180].

In a study of Tarkun et al. [181] in PCOS women and age- and weight-matched healthy women, a comparative analysis of TNF-α and IL-6 was made, with an assessment of their role in IR pathogenesis. Higher concentrations of TNF-α and IL-6 were found in PCOS women compared to controls. A positive correlation was observed between TNF-α and BMI, waist circumference, triglycerides, basal insulin and HOMA-index ($P < 0.001$). IL-6 correlated positively with basal glucose and degree of IR ($P < 0.05$). The authors concluded that TNF-α and IL-6 have a pathogenetic role in the development of IR in PCOS [181].

In another study consisting of obese PCOS women, weight-matched healthy women and normal weight controls Vgontzas et al. [182] determined basal cytokine concentrations and conducted an 8-h nocturnal polysomnography searching for obstructive sleep apnea syndrome. Higher IL-6 plasma concentrations were observed in PCOS women as compared to obese and normal-weight controls (4.75 ± 0.5; 3.65 ± 0.4; 1.84 ± 0.3 pg/mL, respectively, $P < 0.01$). TNF-α levels were somewhat higher in the obese PCOS and control women compared to the normal-weight women, but the differences did not reach statistical significance (4.05 ± 0.3; 3.79 ± 0.2; 3.14 ± 0.2 pg/mL, respectively, $P = 0.103$). IL-6 and TNFα correlated positively with BMI ($P < 0.01$) in the obese healthy women, but not in the obese PCOS women. In addition, a stronger correlation of IL-6 and TNF-α levels with IR indexes (HOMA and QUICKI) was established in the PCOS women than in the obese controls. The authors came to the conclusion that IL-6 may be elevated in PCOS women, irrespectively of obesity and presence of obstructive sleep apnea, and may have a role in the process of IR in this syndrome [182].

Grimaldi Barcellos et al. [183] investigated the impact of PCOS and obesity on the levels of TNFα, IL-6 and CRP in young PCOS women and age- and BMI-matched women with a normal menstrual cycle without CVD risk factors (DM, dyslipidemia, arterial hypertension). The authors did not establish a significant difference in the levels of TNF-α, IL-6 and CRP between the PCOS women and the controls (2.1 *vs* 1.9 pg/mL, $P = 0.397$; 3.8 *vs* 5.7 pg/mL, $P = 0.805$, and 0.9 *vs* 0.5 ng/mL, $P = 0.361$). The TNF-α levels were similar between obese and normal-weight women. IL-6 and CRP were significantly higher in women with overweight/obesity than in normal-weight women (8.7 *vs* 2.0 pg/mL, $P < 0.001$, and 1.4 *vs* 0.2 ng/mL, $P < 0.001$). The authors concluded that obesity, but not PCOS itself, affects the levels of circulating markers of a chronic low-grade inflammation in young carriers of the syndrome without major CVD risk factors [183].

The pathogenesis of an inflammatory process development in MetS, and in particular in PCOS, has not yet been fully clarified. In scientific terms, the most logical and most widespread is the explanation that the higher amount of adipose tissue in case of obesity leads to increased excretion of IL-6 and TNF-α in the circulation, which in turn causes increased production of CRP by the liver. There is another hypothesis highlighting IR as the primary cause of the higher production of cytokines [184].

5. Conclusion

Women with PCOS, combining IR and hyperandrogenism are carriers of an unfavorable cardiovascular risk profile. However, data concerning the long-term risk of cardiovascular morbidity and mortality are scarce, controversial and this issue has not yet been addressed appropriately in targeted large prospective studies. However, since there is compelling evidence of the presence of MetS components and early stages of atherosclerotic processes in young PCOS women that are still reversible, it is essential that they must be diagnosed on the basis of the current knowledge in order to administer adequate complex treatment to prevent late consequences of IR.

Author details

Maria Mitkova Orbetzova
Clinic of Endocrinology and Metabolic Diseases, "Sv. Georgy" University Hospital, Medical University, Plovdiv, Bulgaria

*Address all correspondence to: morbetzova@abv.bg

References

[1] Carmina E, Lobo RA. Polycystic ovary syndrome (PCOS): Arguably the most common endocrinopathy is associated with significant morbidity in women. The Journal of Clinical Endocrinology and Metabolism. 1999;**84**(6):1897-1899

[2] Strauss JF III. Thoughts on the pathophysiology and genetics of polycystic ovary syndrome. Annals of the New York Academy of Sciences. 2003;**997**:42-48

[3] Solomon CG. The epidemiology of polycystic ovary syndrome. Prevalence and associated disease risks. Endocrinology and Metabolism Clinics of North America. 1999;**28**(2):247-263

[4] Moghetti P. Insulin resistance: What is its role in the polycystic ovary syndrome? Current Opinion in Endocrinology & Diabetes. 2002;**9**(6):444-450

[5] Nestler JE. Insulin resistance and the polycystic ovary syndrome: Recent advances. Current Opinion in Endocrinology and Diabetes. 2000;**7**:345-349

[6] Cho LW, Randeva HS, Atkin SL. Cardiometabolic aspects of polycystic ovarian syndrome. Vascular Health and Risk Management. 2007;**3**(1):55-63

[7] Stein IF, Leventhal ML. Amenorrhea associated with bilateral polycystic ovaries. American Journal of Obstetrics and Gynecology. 1935;**29**:181-186

[8] Amowitz LL, Sobel BE. Cardiovascular consequences of polycystic ovary syndrome. Endocrinology and Metabolism Clinics of North America. 1999;**28**:439-458

[9] Dahlgren E, Janson PO, Johansson JS, et al. Polycystic ovary syndrome and risk for myocardial infarction. Evaluated from a risk factor model based on a prospective population study of women. Acta Obstetricia et Gynecologica Scandinavica. 1992;**71**:599-604

[10] Talbott E, Guzick D, Clerici A, et al. Coronary heart disease risk factors in women with polycystic ovary syndrome. Arteriosclerosis, Thrombosis, and Vascular Biology. 1995;**15**(7):821-826

[11] Gambineri A, Pelusi C, Vicennati V, et al. Obesity and the polycystic ovary syndrome. International Journal of Obesity. 2002;**26**:883-896

[12] Mather KJ, Kwan F, Corenblum B. Hyperinsulinemia in polycystic ovary syndrome correlates with increased cardiovascular risk independent of obesity. Fertility and Sterility. 2000;**73**:150-156

[13] Graf MJ, Richards CJ, Brown V, et al. The independent effects of hyperandrogenaemia, hyperinsulinaemia, and obesity on lipid and lipoprotein profiles in women. Clinical Endocrinology. 1990;**33**:119-131

[14] Toscano V, Bianchi P, Balducci R, et al. Lack of linear relationship between hyperinsulinaemia and hyperandrogenism. Clinical Endocrinology. 1992;**36**:197-202

[15] Ciampelli M, Fulghesu AM, Cucinelli F, et al. Impact of insulin and body mass index on metabolic and endocrine variables in polycystic ovary syndrome. Metabolism. 1999;**48**:167-172

[16] Vidal-Puig A, Munoz-Torres M, Jodar-Gimeno E, et al. Hyperinsulinaemia in polycystic ovary syndrome: Relationship to clinical and hormonal factors. The Clinical Investigator. 1994;**72**:853-857

[17] Wild RA. Obesity, lipids, cardiovascular risk, and androgen excess [review]. The American Journal of Medicine. 1995;**98**:27S-32S

[18] Pasquali R, Gambineri A, Anconetani B, et al. The natural history of the metabolic syndrome in young women with the polycystic ovary syndrome and the effect of long-term oestrogen-progestagen treatment. Clinical Endocrinology. 1999;**50**(4):517-527

[19] Orbetzova M. Cardiovascular risk, subclinical and clinically overt cardiovascular diseases in polycystic ovary syndrome. *In* Prevention, Diagnosis, Treatment – Current Problems, 2018; eds. M. Vlaskovska, M. Orbetzova, B. Georgiev, G. Momekov, L. Kirov. Sofia Havitis; pp.445-485 . ISBN: 978-954-92936-0-9 (In Bulgarian)

[20] Dunaif A, Graf M, Mandeli J, et al. Characterization of groups of hyperandrogenic women with acanthosis nigricans, impaired glucose tolerance, and/or hyperinsulinemia. The Journal of Clinical Endocrinology & Metabolism. 1987;**65**:499-507

[21] Legro RS. Diabetes prevalence and risk factors in polycystic ovary syndrome. Current Opinion in Endocrinology & Diabetes. 2002;**9**(6):451-458

[22] Legro RS, Kunselman AR, Dodson WC, et al. Prevalence and predictors of risk for type 2 diabetes mellitus and impaired glucose tolerance in polycystic ovary syndrome: A prospective, controlled study in 254 affected women. The Journal of Clinical Endocrinology and Metabolism. 1999;**84**:165-169

[23] Gambineri A, Pelusi C, Manicardi E, et al. Glucose intolerance in a large cohort of Mediterranean women with polycystic ovary syndrome: phenotype and associated factors. Diabetes. 2004;**53**:2353-2358

[24] Dabadaghao P, Roberts BJ, Wang J, et al. Glucose tolerance abnormalities in Australian women with polycystic ovary syndrome. Medical Journal of Australia. 2007;**187**(6):328-331

[25] Talbott EO, Zborovski JV, Bourdreaux MY. Do women with polycystic ovary syndrome have an increased risk of cardiovascular disease? Review of the evidence. Minerva Ginecologica. 2004;**57**:27-39

[26] Elting MW, Korsen TJ, Bezemer PD, et al. Prevalence of diabetes mellitus, hypertension and cardiac complaints in a follow-up study of a Dutch PCOS population. Human Reproduction. 2001;**16**:556-560

[27] Orbetzova M, Kamenov Z, Kolarov G, et al. Metabolic disturbances in women with polycystic ovary syndrome. Folia Medica. 2003;**3**:12-20

[28] Orbetzova M, Orbetzova V, Kamenov Z, et al. Comparison of the diagnostic indices for evaluation of disorders in carbohydrate metabolism in women with polycystic ovary syndrome (PCOS). Akusherstvo i Ginekologia. 2003;**42**(4):10-15 (in Bulgarian)

[29] Lanzone A, Caruso A, Di Simone N, et al. Polycystic ovary disease. A risk factor for gestational diabetes? The Journal of Reproductive Medicine. 1995;**40**:312-316

[30] Kousta E, Cela E, Lawrence N, et al. The prevalence of polycystic ovaries in women with a history of gestational diabetes. Clinical Endocrinology. 2000;**53**:501-507

[31] Anttila L, Karjala K, Penttila RA, et al. Polycystic ovaries in women with gestational diabetes. Obstetrics and Gynecology. 1998;**92**:13-16

[32] Koivunen RM, Juutinen J, Vauhkonen I, et al. Metabolic and steroidogenic alterations related to

increased frequency of polycystic ovaries in women with a history of ges tational diabetes. Journal of Clinical Endocrinology & Metabolism. 2001;**86**:2591-2599

[33] Conn J, Jacobs HS, Conway GS. The prevalence of polycystic ovaries in women with type 2 diabetes mellitus. Clinical Endocrinology. 2000;**52**:81-86

[34] Burghen GA, Givens JR, Kitabchi AE. Correlation of hyperandrogenism with hyperinsulinism in polycystic ovarian disease. The Journal of Clinical Endocrinology and Metabolism. 1980;**50**:113-116

[35] Dunaif A, Segal KR, Futterweit W, et al. Profound peripheral insulin resistance, independent of obesity, in polycystic ovary syndrome. Diabetes. 1989;**38**:1165-1174

[36] Grulet H, Hecart AC, Delemer B, et al. Roles of LH and insulin resistance in lean and obese polycystic ovary syndrome. Clinical Endocrinology. 1993;**38**:621-626

[37] Chae SJ, Kim JJ, Choi YM, et al. Clinical and biochemical characteristics of polycystic ovary syndrome in Korean women. Human Reproduction. 2008;**23**(8):1924-1931

[38] Holte J, Bergh T, Berne C, et al. Restored insulin sensitivity but persistently increased early insulin secretion after weight loss in obese women with polycystic ovary syndrome. The Journal of Clinical Endocrinology and Metabolism. 1995;**80**(9):2586-2593

[39] Kiddy DS, Hamilton-Fairley D, Bush A, et al. Improvement in endocrine and ovarian function during dietary treatment of obese women with polycystic ovary syndrome. Clinical Endocrinology. 1992;**36**:105-111

[40] Pasquali R, Gambineri A, Biscotti D, et al. Effect of long-term treatment with metformin added to hypocaloric diet on body composition, fat distribution, and androgen and insulin levels in abdominally obese women with and without polycystic ovary syndrome. Journal of Clinical Endocrinology & Metabolism. 2000;**85**:2767-2774

[41] Azziz R, Ehrmann E, Legro RS, et al. Troglitazone improves ovulation and hirsutism in the polycystic ovary syndrome: A multicenter, double blind, placebo-controlled trial. Journal of Clinical Endocrinology & Metabolism. 2001;**86**:1626-1632

[42] Shoupe D, Kumar DD, Lobo RA. Insulin resistance in polycystic ovary syndrome. American Journal of Obstetrics and Gynecology. 1983;**147**:588-592

[43] Dunaif A, Segal KR, Shelley DR, et al. Evidence for distinctive and intrinsic defects in insulin action in polycystic ovary syndrome. Diabetes. 1992;**41**:1257-1266

[44] Holte J, Bergh T, Berne C, et al. Enhanced early insulin response to glucose in relation to insulin resistance in women with polycystic ovary syndrome and normal glucose tolerance. The Journal of Clinical Endocrinology & Metabolism. 1994;**78**:1052-1058

[45] Holte J, Gennarelli G, Berne C, et al. Elevated ambulatory day-time blood pressure in women with polycystic ovary syndrome: A sign of a pre-hypertensive state? Human Reproduction. 1996;**11**(1):23-28

[46] Morales AJ, Laughlin GA, Butzow T, et al. Insulin, somatotropic, and luteinizing hormone axes in lean and obese women with polycystic ovary syndrome: Common and distinct features. The Journal of Clinical Endocrinology and Metabolism. 1996;**81**:2854-2864

[47] Kolarov G, Orbetzova M. Polycystic Ovary Syndrome. Sofia: Viara; 2004. ISBN 954-9409-01-5; 232 pp. (in Bulgarian)

[48] Kamenov Z, Orbetzova M, Gateva A. Polycystic Ovary Syndrome. Sofia: ZIP Ltd.; 2010 258 p. ISBN 978-954-9369-17-5 (in Bulgarian)

[49] Orbetzova M. Polycystic ovary syndrome (PCOS). Epidemiology, pathophysiology, clinical course, complications. Nauka Endokrinologia. 2007;**1**:7-10 (in Bulgarian)

[50] Dunaif A. DT Finegood. Beta-cell dysfunction independent of obesity and glucose intolerance in the polycystic ovary syndrome. The Journal of Clinical Endocrinology and Metabolism. 1996;**81**:942-947

[51] Ehrmann DA, Sturis J, Byrne MM, et al. Insulin secretory defects in polycystic ovary syndrome. Relationship to insulin sensitivity and family history of non-insulin-dependent diabetes mellitus. The Journal of Clinical Investigation. 1995;**96**:520-527

[52] Arslanian SA, Lewy VD, Danadian K. Glucose intolerance in obese adolescents with polycystic ovary syndrome:Roles of insulin resistance and [beta]-cell dysfunction and risk of cardiovascular disease. The Journal of Clinical Endocrinology and Metabolism. 2001;**86**:66-71

[53] Paterakis TS, Diamanti-Kandarakis E. Aspects of cardiometabolic risk in women with polycystic ovary syndrome. Current Obesity Reports. 2014;**3**:377-386

[54] Ciaraldi TP, El-Roeiy A, Madar Z, et al. Cellular mechanism of insulin resistance in polycystic ovarian syndrome. The Journal of Clinical Endocrinology and Metabolism. 1992;**75**:577-583

[55] Rosenbaum D, Haber RS, Dunaif A. Insulin resistance in polycystic ovary syndrome: Decreased expression of GLUT-4 glucose transporters in adipocytes. The American Journal of Physiology. 1993;**264**:E197-E202

[56] El Mkadem SA, Lautier C, Macari F, et al. Role of allelic variants Gly972Arg of IRS-1 and Gly1057Asp of IRS-2 in moderate-to-severe insulin resistance of women with polycystic ovary syndrome. Diabetes. 2001;**50**:2164-2168

[57] Eldar-Geva T, Spitz IM, Groome NP, et al. Follistatin and activin A serum concentrations in obese and non-obese patients with polycystic ovary syndrome. Human Reproduction. 2001;**16**:2552-2556

[58] El-Roeiy A, Chen X, Roberts VJ, et al. Expression of insulin-like growth factor I (IGF-I) and IGF-II and the IGF-I, IGF-II, and insulin receptor genes and localization of the gene products in the human ovary. The Journal of Clinical Endocrinology and Metabolism. 1993;**77**:1411-1518

[59] Suikkari AM, Koivisto VA, Koistinen R, et al. Dose-response characteristics for suppression of low molecular weight plasma insulin-like growth factor-binding protein by insulin. The Journal of Clinical Endocrinology and Metabolism. 1989;**68**:135-140

[60] Zhang LH, Rodriguez H, Ohno S, Miller WL. Serine phosphorylation of human P450c17 increases 17,20-lyase activity: Implications for adrenarche and the polycystic ovary syndrome. Proceedings of the National Academy of Sciences of the United States of America. 1995;**92**:10619-10623

[61] Rosen ED, Spiegelman BM. Tumor necrosis factor-a as a mediator of insulin resistance of obesity. Current Opinion in Endocrinology & Diabetes. 1999;**6**:170-176

[62] Book CB, Dunaif A. Selective insulin resistance in the polycystic

ovary syndrome. The Journal of Clinical Endocrinology and Metabolism. 1999;**84**:3110-3116

[63] Poretsky L, Seto-Young D, Shrestha A, et al. Phosphatidyl-inositol-3 kinase-independent insulin action pathway(s) in the human ovary. The Journal of Clinical Endocrinology and Metabolism. 2001;**86**:3115-3119

[64] Dunaif A, Thomas A. Current concepts in the polycystic ovary syndrome. Annual Review of Medicine. 2001;**52**:401-419

[65] Conway G, Avey C, Rumsby G. The tyrosine kinase domain of the insulin receptor gene is normal in women with hyperinsulinaemia and polycystic ovary syndrome. Human Reproduction. 1994;**9**:1681-1683

[66] Sorbara LR, Tang Z, Cama A, et al. Absence of insulin receptor gene mutations in three insulin-resistant women with the polycystic ovary syndrome. Metabolism, Clinical and Experimental. 1994;**43**:1568-1574

[67] Talbott JA, Bicknell EJ, Rajkhowa M, et al. Molecular scanning of the insulin receptor gene in women with polycystic ovarian syndrome. The Journal of Clinical Endocrinology and Metabolism. 1996;**81**:1979-1983

[68] Ek I, Arner P, Ryden M, et al. A unique defect in the regulation of visceral fat cell lypolysis in the polycystic ovary syndrome as an early link to insulin resistance. Diabetes. 2002;**51**:484-492

[69] Hoffstedt J, Wahrenberg H, Thorne A, et al. The metabolic syndrome is related to beta-adrenoreceptor sensitivity in visceral adipose tissue. Diabetologia. 1996;**39**:838-844

[70] Azziz R, Carmina E, Chen Z, et al. Polycystic ovary syndrome. Nature Reviews Disease Primers. 2016;**2**:16057

[71] Robinson S, Kiddy D, Gelding SV, et al. The relationship of insulin insensitivity to menstrual pattern in women with hyperandrogenism and polycystic ovaries. Clinical Endocrinology. 1993;**39**:351-355

[72] Nestler JE, Strauss JE III. Insulin as an effector of human ovarian and adrenal steroid metabolism. Endocrinology and Metabolism Clinics of North America. 1991;**20**:807-823

[73] Franks S, Mason H, White D, Willis D. Mechanisms of anovulation in polycystic ovary syndrome. In: Flicori M, Flamigni C, editors. The Ovary: Regulation, Dysfunction and Treatment. Amsterdam: Elsevier; 1991. pp. 183-186

[74] White D, Leigh A, Wilson C, Donaldson A, Franks S. Gonadotropin and gonadal steroid response to a single dose of a long-acting agonist of gonadotropin-releasing hormone in ovulatory and anovulatory women with polycystic ovary syndrome. Clinical Endocrinology. 1995;**42**:475-481

[75] Willis DS, Watson H, Mason HD, et al. Premature response to luteinizing hormone of granulosa cells from anovulatory women with polycystic ovary syndrome: Relevance to mechanism of anovulation. The Journal of Clinical Endocrinology and Metabolism. 1998;**83**:3984-3991

[76] Escobar-Morreale HF, Roldan B, Barrio R, et al. High prevalence of the polycystic ovary syndrome and hirsutism in women with type 1 diabetes mellitus. The Journal of Clinical Endocrinology and Metabolism. 2000;**85**:4182-4187

[77] Legro RS, Gnatuk CL, Kunselman AR, Dunaif A. Changes in glucose tolerance over time in women with polycystic ovary syndrome: A controlled study. The Journal of Clinical

Endocrinology and Metabolism. 2005;**90**:3236-3242

[78] Norman RJ, Masters L, Milner CR, et al. Relative risk of conversion from normoglycaemia to impaired glucose tolerance or non-insulin dependent diabetes mellitus in polycystic ovarian syndrome. Human Reproduction. 2001;**16**:1995-1998

[79] Boudreaux MY, Talbott EO, Kip KE, et al. Risk of T2DM and impaired fasting glucose among PCOS subjects: Results of an 8-year follow-up. Current Diabetes Reports. 2006;**6**:77-83

[80] Livadas S, Kollias A, Panidis D, Diamanti-Kandarakis E. Diverse impacts of aging on insulin resistance in lean and obese women with polycystic ovary syndrome: Evidence from 1345 women with the syndrome. European Journal of Endocrinology. 2014;**171**:301-309

[81] Moghetti P, Tosi F, Bonin C, et al. Divergences in insulin resistance between the different phenotypes of the polycystic ovary syndrome. The Journal of Clinical Endocrinology and Metabolism. 2013;**98**:E628-E637

[82] Bil E, Dilbaz B, Cirik DA, et al. Metabolic syndrome and metabolic risk profile according to polycystic ovary syndrome phenotype. The Journal of Obstetrics and Gynaecology Research. 2016;**42**:837-843

[83] AACE - American Association of Clinical Endocrinologists. Position statement on metabolic and cardiovascular consequences of polycystic ovary syndrome. Endocrine practice. 2005;**11**(2):125-134

[84] Ehrmann DA. Polycystic ovary syndrome. The New England Journal of Medicine. 2005;**352**(12):1223-1236

[85] Carmina E, Koyama T, Chang L, et al. Does ethnicity influence the prevalence of adrenal hyperandrogenism and insulin resistance in polycystic ovary syndrome? American Journal of Obstetrics and Gynecology. 1992;**167**(06):1807-1812

[86] Carmina E, Legro RS, Stamets K, et al. Difference in body weight between American and Italian women with polycystic ovary syndrome: Influence of the diet. Human Reproduction. 2003;**18**(11):2289-2293

[87] Lim SS, Davies MJ, Norman RJ, Moran LJ. Overweight, obesity and central obesity in women with polycystic ovary syndrome: A systematic review and meta-analysis. Human Reproduction Update. 2012;**18**(06):618-637

[88] Lizneva D, Kirubakaran R, Mykhalchenko K, et al. Phenotypes and body mass in women with polycystic ovary syndrome identified in referral versus unselected populations: Systematic review and meta-analysis. Fertility and Sterility. 2016;**106**(06):1510-1520

[89] Lizneva D, Suturina L, Walker W, et al. Criteria, prevalence, and phenotypes of polycystic ovary syndrome. Fertility and Sterility. 2016;**106**(01):6-15

[90] Diamanti-Kandarakis E, Kouli CR, Bergiele AT, et al. A survey of the polycystic ovary syndrome in the Greek island of Lesbos: Hormonal and metabolic profile. The Journal of Clinical Endocrinology and Metabolism. 1999;**84**:4006-4011

[91] Orbetzova M. Polycystic ovary syndrome. In: Vlaskovska M, Tankova T, Popova D, Georgiev B, editors. Prophylaxis, Diagnostics, Therapy - Current Problems 2012. Sofia: Havitis; 2012. pp. 407-434. ISBN: 978-954-92936-1-6 (in Bulgarian)

[92] Godoy-Matos AF, Vaisman F, Pedrosa AP, et al. Central-to-peripheral

fat ratio, but not peripheral body fat, is related to insulin resistance and androgen markers in polycystic ovary syndrome. Gynecological Endocrinology. 2009;**25**:793-798

[93] Strowitzki T, Halser B, Demant T. Body fat distribution, insulin sensitivity, ovarian dysfunction and serum lipoproteins in patients with polycystic ovary syndrome. Gynecological Endocrinology. 2002;**16**:45-51

[94] Cosar E, Üçok K, Akgün L, et al. Body fat composition and distribution in women with polycystic ovary syndrome. Gynecological Endocrinology. 2008;**24**:428-432

[95] Liou T-H, Yang J-H, Hsieh C-H, et al. Clinical and biochemical presentations of polycystic ovary syndrome among obese and nonobese women. Fertility and Sterility. 2009;**92**:1960-1965

[96] Kiddy DS, Sharp PS, White DM, et al. Differences in clinical and endocrine features between obese and non-obese subjects with polycystic ovary syndrome: An analysis of 263 consecutive cases. Clinical Endocrinology. 1990;**32**:213-220

[97] Karabulut A, Yaylali GF, Demirlenk S, et al. Evaluation of body fat distribution in PCOS and its association with carotid atherosclerosis and insulin resistance. Gynecological Endocrinology. 2012;**28**:111-114

[98] Conway GS, Agrawal R, Betteridge DJ, Jacobs HS. Risk factors for coronary artery disease in lean and obese women with the polycystic ovary syndrome. Clinical Endocrinology. 1992;**37**:119-125

[99] Svendsen PF, Nilas L, Norgaard K, et al. Obesity, body composition and metabolic disturbances in polycystic ovary syndrome. Human Reproduction. 2008;**23**:2113-2121

[100] Cree-Green M, Rahat H, Newcomer B, Bergman B. Insulin resistance, hyperinsulinemia and mitochondria dysfunction in non-obese girls with polycystic ovary syndrome. Journal of the Endocrine Society. 2017;**1**:931-944

[101] Thaler MA, Seifert-Klauss V, Luppa PB. The biomarker sex hormone-binding globulin – From established applications to emerging trends in clinical medicine. Best Practice & Research Clinical Endocrinology & Metabolism. 2015;**29**:749-760

[102] Sutton-Tyrrell K, Wildman RP, Matthews KA, et al. Sex hormone-binding globulin and the free androgen index are related to cardiovascular risk factors in multiethnic premenopausal and perimenopausal women enrolled in the study of women across the nation (SWAN). Circulation. 2005;**111**:1242-1249

[103] Milcheva B, Orbetzova M. Adipose tissue – endocrine organ. Endocrinologia. 2004;**9**(2):64-72 (in Bulgarian)

[104] Orbetzova M. Adipose-tissue hormones at women with polycystic ovary syndrome. Literature review with own data. Nauka Endokrinologia. 2009;**6**:258-261 (in Bulgarian)

[105] Calvar CE, Intebi AD, Bengolea SV, et al. Leptin in patients with polycystic ovary syndrome. Direct correlation with insulin resistance. Medicina B Aires. 2003;**63**:704-710

[106] Morin-Papunen L, Koivunen R, Tomas C, et al. Decreased serum leptin concentrations during metformin therapy in obese women with polycystic ovary syndrome. The Journal of Clinical Endocrinology and Metabolism. 1998;**83**:2566-2568

[107] Orbetzova M, Pehlivanov B, Mitkov M, et al. Effect of short-term

standard therapeutic regimens on neuropeptide Y and adipose tissue hormones in overweight Insulinresistant women with polycystic ovary syndrome. Folia Medica. 2011;**53**(3):15-24

[108] Koleva DI, Orbetzova MM, Atanassova PK. Adipose tissue hormones and appetite and body weight regulators in insulin resistance. Folia Medica. 2013;**55**(1):25-32

[109] Koleva DI. Adipose tissue hormones, appetite and body weight regulators, and endothelial function in women with insulin resistance. Abstract of a doctoral thesis for the award of educational and scientific degree "PhD". Plovdiv; 2017 (in Bulgarian)

[110] Mohiti-Ardekani J, Tarof N, Aflatonian A. Relationships between free leptin and insulin resistance in women with polycystic ovary syndrome. Iranian Journal of Reproductive Medicine. 2009;7(2):53-58

[111] Chapman IM, Wittert GA, Norman RJ. Circulating leptin concentrations in polycystic ovary syndrome: Relation to anthropometric and metabolic parameters. Clinical Endocrinology. 1997;**46**:175-181

[112] Spritzer PM, Poy M, Wiltgen D, et al. Leptin concentrations in hirsute women with polycystic ovary syndrome or idiopathic hirsutism: Influence on LH and relationship with hormonal, metabolic, and anthropometric measurements. Human Reproduction. 2001;**16**:1340-1346

[113] Pirwany IR, Fleming R, Sattar N, et al. Circulating leptin concentrations and ovarian function in polycystic ovary syndrome. European Journal of Endocrinology. 2001;**145**:289-294

[114] Rouru J, Anttila L, Koskinen P, et al. Serum leptin concentrations in women with polycystic ovary syndrome. The Journal of Clinical Endocrinology and Metabolism. 1997;**82**:1697-1700

[115] Carmina E, Ferin M, Gonzalez F, et al. Evidence that insulin and androgens may participate in the regulation of serum leptin levels in women. Fertility and Sterility. 1999;**72**:926-931

[116] Gennarelli G, Holte J, Wide L, et al. Is there a role for leptin in the endocrine and metabolic aberrations of polycystic ovary syndrome? Human Reproduction. 1998;**13**:535-541

[117] Telli MH, Yildirim M, Noyan V. Serum leptin levels in patients with polycystic ovary syndrome. Fertility and Sterility. 2002;**77**:932-935

[118] Mantzorous CS, Dunaif A, Fiiler S. Leptin concentration in the polysistic ovary syndroume. The Journal of Clinical Endocrinology and Metabolism. 1997;**82**:1697-1700

[119] Laughlin GA, Morales AJ, Yen SS. Serum leptin levels in women with polycystic ovary syndrome: The role of insulin resistance/hyperinsulinemia. The Journal of Clinical Endocrinology and Metabolism. 1997;**82**:1692-1696

[120] Nomair AM, Aref NK, Rizwan F, et al. Serum leptin level in obese women with polycystic ovary syndrome, and its relation to insulin resistance. Asian Pacific Journal of Reproduction. 2014;**3**(4):288-294

[121] Pittas AG, Joseph NA, Greenberg AS. Adipocytokines and insulin resistance. The Journal of Clinical Endocrinology and Metabolism. 2004;**89**(2):447-452

[122] Kadowaki T, Yamauchi T. Adiponectin and adiponectin receptors. Endocrine Reviews. 2005;**26**(3):439-451

[123] Orbetzova M, Atanasova I, Milcheva B, et al. Adiponectin and its

relation to certain clinical, hormonal and metabolic characteristics at women with android obesity. Endocrinologia. 2007;**1**:4-17 (in Bulgarian)

[124] Reinhart RA, Gani K, Arndt MR, et al. Apolipoproteins AI and B as predictors of angiographically defined coronary artery disease. Archives of Internal Medicine. 1990;**150**(8):1629-1633

[125] Hu E, Liang P, Spiegelman BM. AdipoQ is a novel adipose-specific gene dysregulated in obesity. The Journal of Biological Chemistry. 1996;**271**:10697-10703

[126] Yamamoto Y, Hirose H, Saito I, et al. Correlation of the adipocyte-derived protein adiponectin with insulin resistance index and serum high-density lipoprotein-cholesterol, independent of body mass index, in the Japanese population. Clinical Science. 2002;**103**:137-142

[127] Weyer C, Funahashi T, Tanaka S, et al. Hypoadiponectinemia in obesity and type 2 diabetes: Close association with insulin resistance and hyperinsulinemia. The Journal of Clinical Endocrinology and Metabolism. 2001;**86**:1930-1935

[128] Orio F, Palomba S, Kascella T, et al. Adiponectin levels in women with polycystic ovary syndrome. The Journal of Clinical Endocrinology and Metabolism. 2003;**88**:2619-2623

[129] Panidis D, Kourtis A, Farmakiotis D, et al. Serum adiponectin levels in women with polycystic ovary syndrome. Human Reproduction. 2003;**18**(9):1790-1796

[130] Sepilan V, Nagamani M. Adiponectin levels in women with polycystic ovary syndrome and severe insulin resistance. Journal of the Society for Gynecologic Investigation. 2005;**12**(2):129-134

[131] Koleva DI, Orbetzova MM, Nyagolova PV, Mitkov MD. Adipokines, metabolic and atherogenic parameters in insulin resistant and non-insulin resistant women with polycystic ovary syndrome. Giornale Italiano di Ostetricia e Ginecologia. 2016;**38**(1):114-118

[132] Norata GD, Raselli S, Grigore L, et al. Leptin: Adiponectin ratio is an independent predictor of intima media thickness of the common carotid artery. Stroke. 2007;**38**:2844-2846

[133] Filippidis G, Liakopoulos V, Mertens PR, et al. Resistin serum levels are increased but not correlated with insulin resistance in chronic hemodialysis patients. Blood Purification. 2005;**23**:421-428

[134] Azuma K, Katsukawa F, Oguchi S, et al. Correlation between serum resistin level and adiposity in obese individuals. Obesity Research. 2003;**11**(8):997-1001

[135] Orbetzova M, Atanassova I, Milcheva B, et al. Adipose tissue hormones in women with different morphotypes of overweight. Endocrinologia. 2004;**9**(4):214-224 (In Bulgarian)

[136] Lee JH, Chan JL, Yiannakouris N, et al. Circulating resistin levels are not associated with obesity or insulin resistance in humans and are not regulated by fasting or leptin administration: Cross-sectional and interventional studies in normal, insulinresistant, and diabetic subjects. The Journal of Clinical Endocrinology and Metabolism. 2003;**88**(10):4848-4856

[137] Silha JV, Krsek M, Skrha JV. Plasma resistin, adiponectin and leptin levels in lean and o bese subjects: Correlations with insulin resistance. European Journal of Endocrinology. 2003;**149**(4):331-335

[138] Carmina E, Orio F, Palomba S, et al. Endothelial dysfunction in PCOS:

Role of obesity and adipose hormones. The American Journal of Medicine. 2006;**119**:356-366

[139] Panidis D, Koliakos G, Kourtis A, et al. Serum resistin levels in women with polycystic ovary syndrome. Fertility and Sterility. 2004;**81**(2):361-366

[140] Munir I, Yen HW, Baruth T, et al. Resistin stimulation of 17 alpha hydroxylase activity in ovarian theca cells in vitro: Relevance to polycystic ovary synd Rome. The Journal of Clinical Endocrinology and Metabolism. 2005;**90**:4852-4857

[141] Pangaribuan B, Yusuf I, Mansyur M, et al. Serum adiponectin and resistin in relation to insulin resistance and markers of hyperandrogenism in lean and obese women with polycystic ovary syndrome. Therapeutic Advances in Endocrinology and Metabolism. 2011;**2**(6):235-245

[142] Seow KM, Juan CC, Wu LY, et al. Serum and adipocyte resistin in polycystic ovary syndrome with insulin resistance. Human Reproduction. 2004;**19**(1):48-53

[143] Olszanecka-Glinianowicz M, Kuglin D, Dąbkowska-Huć A, et al. Serum adiponectin and resistin in relation to insulin resistance and markers of hyperandrogenism in lean and obese women with polycystic ovary syndrome. European Journal of Obstetrics, Gynecology, and Reproductive Biology. 2011;**154**(1):51-56

[144] Lewandowski KC, Szosland K, O'Callaghan C, et al. Adiponectin and resistin serum levels in women with polycystic ovary syndrome during oral glucose tolerance test: A significant reciprocal correlation between adiponectin and resistin independent of insulin resistance indices. Molecular Genetics and Metabolism. 2005;**85**:61-69

[145] Yilmaz M, Bukan N, Demirci H, et al. Serum resistin and adiponectin levels in women with polycystic ovary syndrome. Gynecological Endocrinology. 2009;**25**(4):246-252

[146] Koleva DI, Orbetzova MM, Nyagolova PV, et al. Resistin and insulin resistance in women with polycystic ovary syndrome. Endocrinologia. 2016;**XXI**(4):211-222

[147] Wang Y, Xie X, Zhu W. Serum adiponectin and resistin levels in patients with polycystic ovarian syndrome and their clinical implications. Journal of Huazhong University of Science and Technology. Medical Sciences. 2010;**30**(5):638-642

[148] Kaser S, Kaser A, Sandhofer A, et al. Resistin messenger-RNA expression is increased by proinflammatory cytokines in vitro. Biochemical and Biophysical Research Communications. 2003;**309**:286-290

[149] Malo E, Ukkola O, Jokela M, et al. Resistin is an indicator of the metabolic syndrome according to five different definitions in the Finnish health 2000 survey. Metabolic Syndrome and Related Disorders. 2011;**9**:203-210

[150] Makni E, Moalla W, Benezzeddine-Boussaidi L, et al. Correlation of resistin with inflammatory and cardiometabolic markers in obese adolescents with and without metabolic syndrome. Obesity Facts. 2013;**6**:393-404

[151] Rabe K, Lehrke M, Parhofer KG, et al. Adipokines and insulin resistance. Molecular Medicine. 2008;**14**(11-12):7417-7451

[152] Fukuhara A, Matsuda M, Nishizawa M, et al. A protein secreted by visceral fat that mimics the effects of insulin. Science. 2005;**307**:426-430

[153] Sun Y, Wu Z, Wei L, et al. High visfatin levels in women with polycystic ovary syndrome: Evidence from a meta-analysis. Gynecological Endocrinology. 2015;**31**(10):808-814

[154] Kowalska I, Straczkowski M, Nikolajuk A, et al. Serum visfatin in relation to insulin resistance and markers of hyperandrogenism in lean and obese women with polycystic ovary syndrome. Human Reproduction. 2007;**22**(7):1824-1829

[155] Haider DG, Schaller G, Kapiotis S, et al. The release of the adipocytokine visfatin is regulated by glucose and insulin. Diabetologia. 2006;**49**:1909-1914

[156] Tan B, Chen J, Digby J, et al. Icreased visfatin messenger ribonucleic acid and protein levels in adipose tissue and adipocytes in women with polycystic ovary syndrome: Parallel increase in plasma visfatin. Journal of Clinical Endocrinology and Metabolism. 2006;**91**(12):5022-5028

[157] El-Said MH, El-Said NH, Mohamad NAE-G. Plasma Visfatin concentrations in polycystic ovary syndrome: Relationships with indices of insulin resistance and hyperandrogenism. Medical Journal Cairo University. 2009;**77**(3):1-7

[158] Gen R, Akbay E, Muşlu N, et al. Plasma visfatin level in lean women with PCOS: Relation to proinflammatory markers and insulin resistance. Gynecological Endocrinology. 2009;**25**(4):241-245

[159] Fernarndez-Real JM, Pickup JC. Innate immunity, insulin resistance and type 2 diabetes. Trends in Endocrinology and Metabolism. 2008;**19**:10-16

[160] Moller DE. Potential role of TNF-α in the pathogenesis of insulin resistance and type 2 diabetes. Trends in Endocrinology and Metabolism. 2000;**11**:212-217

[161] Hube F, Birgel M, Hauner H, et al. Expression pattern of tumor necrosis factor receptors im subcutaneous and omental human adipose tissue: Role of obesity and non-insulin dependent diabetes mellitus. European Journal of Clinical Investigation. 1999;**29**:672-678

[162] Kern P, Ranganathan S, Li C. Adipose tissue tumor necrosis factor and interleukin 6 expression in human obesity and insulin resistance. The American Journal of Physiology - Endocrinology and Metabolism. 2001;**280**:E745-E751

[163] Lofgren P, van Harmelen V, Reynisdottir S. Secretion of tumor necrosis factor D shows a strong relationship to insulin stimulated glucose transport in human adipose tissue. Diabetes. 2000;**49**:688-692

[164] Pincelli AI, Brunani A, Scacchi M, et al. The serum concentration of tumor necrosis factor alpha is not an index of growthhormone- or obesity-induced insulin resistance. Hormone Research. 2001;**55**(2):57-64

[165] Bastard JP, Maachi M, Lagathu C, et al. Recent advances in the relationship between obesity, inflammation, and insulin resistance. European Cytokine Network. 2006;**17**:4-12

[166] Araya AV, Aguirre A, Romero C, et al. Evaluation of tumor necrosis factor alpha production in ex vivo short term cultured whole blood from women with polycystic ovary syndrome. European Cytokine Network. 2002;**13**(4):419-424

[167] Gonzalez F, Thusu K, Abdel-Rahman E, et al. Elevated serum levels of tumor necrosis factor alpha in normal-weight women with polycystic ovary syndrome. Metabolism, Clinical and Experimental. 1999;**48**(4):437-441

[168] Soares GM, Vieira CS, Martins WP, et al. Increased arterial stiffness in nonobese women with polycystic ovary syndrome (PCOS) without comorbidities: One more characteristic inherent to the syndrome? Clinical Endocrinology. 2009;**71**:406-411

[169] Mooney RA. Counterpoint: Interleukin-6 does not have a beneficial role in insulin sensitivity and glucose homeostasis. Journal of Applied Physiology. 2007;**102**:816-818

[170] Lin YS, Tsai SJ, Lin MW, et al. Interleukin-6 as an early chronic inflammatory marker in polycystic ovary syndrome with insulin receptor substrate-2 polymorphism. American Journal of Reproductive Immunology. 2011;**66**:527-533

[171] Ibanez L, Valls C, Marcos MV, et al. Insulin sensitization for girls with precocious pubarche and with risk for polycystic ovary syndrome: Effects of prepubertal initiation and postpubertal discontinuation of metformin treatment. The Journal of Clinical Endocrinology and Metabolism. 2004;**89**:4331-4337

[172] Tumu VR, Govatati S, Guruvaiah P, et al. An interleukin-6 gene promoter polymorphism is associated with polycystic ovary syndrome in South Indian women. Journal of Assisted Reproduction and Genetics. 2013;**30**:1541-1546

[173] Ojeda-Ojeda M, Murri M, Insenser M, et al. Mediators of low-grade chronic inflammation in polycystic ovary syndrome (PCOS). Current Pharmaceutical Design. 2013;**19**:5775-5791

[174] Mohlig M, Spranger J, Osterhoff M, et al. The polycystic ovary syndrome per se is not associated with increased chronic inflammation. European Journal of Endocrinology. 2004;**150**:525-532

[175] Escobar-Morreale HF, Villuendas G, Botella-Carretero JI, et al. Obesity, and not insulin resistance, is the major determinant of serum inflammatory cardiovascular risk markers in pre-menopausal women. Diabetologia. 2003;**46**:625-633

[176] Fishman D, Faulds G, Jeffery R, et al. The effect of novel polymorphisms in the interleukin-6 (IL-6) gene on IL-6 transcription and plasma IL-6 levels, and an association with systemic-onset juvenile chronic arthritis. The Journal of Clinical Investigation. 1998;**102**:1369-1376

[177] Hulkkonen J, Pertovaara M, Antonen J, et al. Elevated interleukin-6 plasma levels are regulated by the promoter region polymorphism of the IL-6 gene in primary Sjogren's syndrome and correlate with the clinical manifestations of the disease. Rheumatology. 2001;**40**:656-661

[178] Jones KG, Brull DJ, Brown LC, et al. Interleukin-6 (IL-6) and the prognosis of abdominal aortic aneurysms. Circulation. 2001;**103**:2260-2265

[179] Villuendas G, Millan JLS, Sancho J, Escobar-Morreale HF. The 597 G A and 174 G C polymorphisms in the promoter of the IL-6 gene are associated with hyperandrogenism. The Journal of Clinical Endocrinology & Metabolism. 2002;**87**:1134-1141

[180] Kelly CC, Lyall H, Petrie JR, et al. Low grade chronic inflammation in women with polycystic ovarian syndrome. The Journal of Clinical Endocrinology and Metabolism. 2001;**86**:2453-2455

[181] Tarkun I, Çetinarslan B, Türemen E, et al. Association between circulating tumor necrosis factor-α, interleukin-6, and insulin resistance in normal-weight women with polycystic ovary syndrome. Metabolic Syndrome and Related Disorders. 2006;**4**(2):122-128

[182] Vgontzas AN, Trakada G, Bixler EO, et al. Plasma interleukin 6 levels are elevated in polycystic ovary syndrome independently of obesity or sleep apnea. Metabolism. 2006;**55**(8):1076-1082

[183] Grimaldi Barcellos CR, Rocha MP, Hayashida SAY, et al. Obesity, but not polycystic ovary syndrome, affects circulating markers of low-grade inflammation in young women without major cardiovascular risk factors. Hormones. 2015;**14**(2):251-257

[184] Dandona P, Aljada A, Chaudhuri A, et al. Metabolic syndrome: A comprehensive perspective based on interactions between obesity, diabetes, and inflammation. Circulation. 2005;**111**:1448-1454

Chapter 3

Effects of Exercise Intervention on the Improvement of Polycystic Ovary Syndrome

Shaobing Wang, Zhenghong Zhang and Yiping Liu

Abstract

Polycystic ovary syndrome (PCOS) is a complex endocrine and metabolic disease characterized by hyperandrogenism and insulin resistance. It results in irregular menstruation, obesity and even infertility, which influences badly physical and mental health of the patients. Now, there is no effective drug for treating PCOS and the preferred program is lifestyle modification, including diet control, regular exercise and behavior therapy. Therefore, in the review, we summarize the study progress concerning the effects of lifestyle intervention on the metabolic, reproductive and psychological dysfunctions of PCOS patients and analyze the corresponding mechanisms in these processes. It can radically reduce the factors of PCOS occurrence and development, while providing valuable information for the prevention and treatment of PCOS and is helpful for further research.

Keywords: polycystic ovary syndrome, physiopathology, exercise, lifestyle intervention

1. Introduction

PCOS was an endocrine disorder with complex pathogenesis and diverse clinical phenotypes and was also the most common cause of infertility and abnormal menstrual cycle in women of childbearing age. Current epidemiological investigation showed that PCOS affects 5–10% of women of reproductive age [1]. The effects run through the patient's entire reproductive cycle, from puberty until after menopause, even involving the offspring. PCOS affected patients' reproductive functions, caused of glucose and lipid metabolism disorders, increased the risk of type 2 diabetes and cardiovascular diseases, but also caused anxiety, depression and other psychosocial disorders. Therefore, PCOS was a clinical problem and also a public health problem that needs to be solved urgently [2, 3]. In addition to traditional psychological and drug therapy, exercise had obvious curative effect as a simple and economical adjunctive therapy. In the review, to treat PCOS patients with metabolic, reproductive and psychological dysfunctions, we explored how exercise or combination with other methods could effectively intervene PCOS patients. It provided theoretical basis for clinical treatment of PCOS patients.

2. Exercise or combination with other methods improve reproductive dysfunction in PCOS patients

PCOS accompanied with various clinical manifestations such as obesity, irregular ovulation or anovulation, infertility, menstrual disorder and excessive androgen, insulin resistance and so on. Obese PCOS women showed decreasing reproductive function and increasing risk of metabolic syndrome, but also their mental health and life quality were greatly affected. Before assisted reproduction, weigh loss through diet or exercise therapy and other lifestyle interventions could help restore spontaneous ovulation, increase natural pregnancy rate, improve pregnancy rate and live birth rate of assisted pregnancy, reduce the risk of pregnancy complications, and improve pregnancy outcome.

Current clinical statistics showed that nearly 50% of PCOS patients were associated with obesity [4]. The subcutaneous fat distribution of triceps brachii and subscapular in PCOS patients was significantly different from that in the healthy control group, and the waist-hip ratio (WHR) was significantly higher than that in the control group [5]. PCOS patients were often accompanied by abdominal obesity and visceral fat accumulation. Case control analysis showed that the overall fat content and visceral fat content of PCOS women were significantly higher than that of healthy women, especially abdominal and mesenteric fat [6]. Obesity had a great impact on reproductive health, such as ovulation disorders, decreased pregnancy rate and increased abortion rate, increased risk of pregnancy complications including preeclampsia and gestational diabetes, in addition, when assisted reproductive technology (ART) assisted pregnancy, the response of obese PCOS patients to assisted pregnancy drugs reduced, and the success rate of assisted pregnancy decreased [7].

Lin and Lujan [8] reviewed the diet and exercise of PCOS women and found that there was no significant difference in exercise amount between PCOS women and healthy women, but PCOS women were characterized by high-calorie diet, excessive intake of saturated fatty acid and lack of dietary fiber. After receiving ART assisted pregnancy therapy, the clinical pregnancy rate and live birth rate of obese PCOS women were significantly lower than those of normal weight PCOS patients, and the risk of miscarriage was increased [9, 10]. Therefore, it was very important to control BMI in the optimal range before pregnancy assistance to improve the success rate of ART. For PCOS women aged 25–35 years, BMI should be controlled below 24 kg/m^2. Adjusting the BMI of older women should be more strict and for those over 35 years old, it should be less than 20 kg/m^2 [11]. Obese PCOS patients could lose weight through lifestyle adjustment such as diet, exercise and behavioral intervention to achieve better pregnancy outcome.

2.1 Effects of regular exercise on the pregnancy outcome of PCOS patients

Although the pathogenesis of PCOS was not clear and clinical phenotypes were diverse, PCOS patients with any phenotype may have insulin resistance, with an incidence of 50–80% [12]. More and more evidences showed that insulin resistance was closely related to PCOS. Endocrine disorders caused by genetic environment and obesity were regarded as the cornerstone of PCOS, and insulin resistance was likely to be the initiation factor and central link of PCOS development [13]. Insulin resistance referred to the decrease of the sensitivity of peripheral tissues to insulin, which leading to the decrease of the biological function of insulin and further caused hyperinsulinemia in peripheral blood circulation. Hyperinsulinemia and insulin resistance played various roles in different tissues in the body and promoted the occurrence of hyperandrogenemia. Firstly, on the surface of ovary, acted on insulin-like growth factor binding protein and up-regulated the activity of cytochrome P450c17 alpha enzyme in follicular membrane cells, accelerated the biosynthesis of androgens and promoted the proliferation of follicular membrane cells. Secondly, enhanced the effect of adrenocortical hormone and promoted the production of adrenogenic androgen. Thirdly, in the liver, inhibited the activity of sex hormone-binding globulin (SHBG) and led to increase the levels of free androgen in the blood [14]. Under the action of aromatase in fat cells, excessive androgen converted into a high level of estrogen in the blood and positive feedback to the hypothalamus, kept LH at a high level for a long time. Insulin resistance, hyperandrogen and hypothalamic-pituitary-gonadal axis disorders eventually affected follicular maturation, leading to ovulation disorders, which cause infertility and menstrual cycle disorders.

At present, the international Androgen Excess and PCOS Society (AEPCOS) suggested that physical exercise of more than 150 min per week was recommended to maintain a healthy body quality and condition, including at least 90 min of moderate-high intensity exercise (heart rate 150 times/min), such as football, basketball and other team sports or brisk walking, running, rowing, etc. It is proved that physical exercise could effectively improve menstrual disorders and thin ovulation of obese PCOS patients. It had even been reported that exercise therapy was more beneficial to patients' reproductive function than low-calorie diet therapy. In fact, for obese PCOS patients without ovulation, exercise therapy could restore the regular menstrual cycle in 60% of patients, ovulation in 50% of patients and spontaneously conceive in 35% of patients [15]. Before or in conjunction with medication, exercise intervention could effectively improve health-related life quality of overweight or obese PCOS patients, which can improve the insulin resistance of the patients and help them to increase ovulation rate and decrease hormone level for increasing pregnancy rate [16, 17].

Regular exercise may alleviate insulin resistance of PCOS patients by the two ways. First of all, regular physical exercise could lose weight and significantly reduce visceral fat of PCOS patients. Visceral fat had stronger metabolic activity and was closely related to insulin resistance. Secondly, physical exercise could regulate the expression of insulin signaling protein in skeletal muscle, so as to improve the metabolic level of muscle cells and increased the sensitivity of insulin in PCOS patients.

2.2 Lifestyle adjustment improve the pregnancy outcome of obese PCOS women

Lifestyle and behavioral interventions for weight control required weight loss with regular exercise and diet interventions, as well as long-term target weight maintenance after weight loss. AEPCOS recommended at least 150 min of exercise per week for obese PCOS patients, the sport types included fast walking, jogging, aerobics, swimming and other whole-body exercises involving more than 2/3 of the muscles, the exercise intensity reached medium and high intensity. Heymsfield and Wadden [18] reviewed the mechanism of obesity, pathophysiology and weight loss management and concluded that lifestyle intervention to reduce weight through diet and exercise combined with cognitive behavioral therapy could improve health and quality of life by 5–10% in overweight/obese patients. Cognitive behavioral intervention required professional guidance and could effectively guide diet and exercise by providing encouragement, setting weight loss goals and guiding problems encountered during lifestyle interventions. Regular cognitive behavioral intervention was the most effective way to achieve weight loss and long-term weight maintenance. However, the current problem is that it is difficult to achieve long-term behavioral intervention counseling, resulting in easy weight regain after weight loss. Evidence-based medicine supported PCOS patients to adjust their lifestyle to lose weight, which was helpful to prevent overweight and obesity and improve the long-term quality of life. For PCOS patients of normal weight, there was still a risk of long-term weight gain, so lifestyle intervention was also required. PCOS patients to conduct regular self-monitoring, combine lifestyle intervention with psychological strategies, and developed clinically feasible and economical intervention strategies. Patients with normal weight PCOS received low-intensity interventions to maintain weight and prevent weight gain.

Weight loss therapy included diet, exercise and other lifestyle interventions, weight loss medication and weight loss surgery. As a non-drug intervention, low-calorie diet and exercise with weight loss had strong feasibility, relatively low cost and large benefits. When the weight of obese PCOS women drops by 5%, spontaneous ovulation could be improved and the natural pregnancy rate could be increased [7]. In addition, lifestyle adjustment was beneficial to improve endocrine function, cardiovascular and mental health [19]. Therefore, it was of great significance for overweight/obese PCOS women to help them adjust their lifestyle to reduce weight before pregnancy. It was reported that rapid weight loss had an adverse effect on the outcome of ART assisted pregnancy [20]. Therefore, it was very important to maintain reasonable and stable weight loss and keep long-term weight control, which is also a big problem of obesity PCOS weight loss.

For obese women with endocrine disorders, menoxenia and infertility, adjusting lifestyle to reduce weight was beneficial to improve endocrine function, restore ovulation and increase pregnancy rate. Only 5–10% of weight loss could benefit infertility patients [21–25]. Obese PCOS patients could reduce concentric obesity and improve insulin resistance by adjusting their lifestyle, which was conducive to the recovery of ovulation [26]. A prospective pilot study suggested that lifestyle intervention for weight loss could improve the ovulation function of obese PCOS women. The researchers recruited 32 obese PCOS women with anovulation and conducted lifestyle intervention for 6 months. Compared with the control group of 18 subjects who did not resume ovulation after weight loss by lifestyle intervention, 14 ones of restoring ovulation lost significant weight and significantly reduced abdominal fat. Further analysis found that the reduction of abdominal fat in the ovulation restoration group was more significant than that in the non-ovulation restoration group after lifestyle intervention for 3 and 6 months. It suggested that weight loss and abdominal fat reduction, especially the early and continuous reduction of intra-abdominal fat, was conducive to the recovery of spontaneous ovulation, thereby ultimately improving the natural pregnancy rate [27]. A prospective study by Salama et al. convened 75 overweight/obese PCOS women and implemented a low-calorie diet and exercise intervention for 12 weeks. A total of 27 of the 43 PCOS women with anovulatory amenorrhea resumed their menstrual cycles and seven of the 58 PCOS women had natural pregnancies [28].

For obese PCOS women with fertility requirements, lifestyle intervention and reasonable weight reduction could help improve pregnancy outcome before assisted pregnancy therapy. PCOS patients were often accompanied by androgen overload, irregular ovulation and menstrual disorders. Patients with indications often need to use Oral contraceptive pills (OCP) to adjust menstrual cycle and endocrine function. Legro et al. [29] designed a randomized controlled trial, which 149 overweight/obese infertile PCOS women were pretreated with lifestyle, oral contraceptives or a combination of both for 16 weeks before entering the clomiphene ovulatory cycle to analyze the impact of lifestyle interventions on pregnancy-assisted outcomes. The results indicated that before assisted reproduction, lifestyle interventions combined with oral contraceptives could eliminate the metabolic side effects of oral contraceptives alone. In addition, the ovulation rate and the live birth rate were higher in the lifestyle adjustment or combination with OCP groups than in the OCP group, but there was no significant difference in clinical pregnancy rate between the groups. Legro et al. [30] also conducted secondary analysis on two multi-center clinical trials, overweight or obese infertile PCOS women were pre-treated with lifestyle, oral contraceptives or a combination of both before entering the clomiphene ovulation cycle. In this study, subjects who entered the ovulation induction cycle without any preconditioning were used as the control group, and the assisted pregnancy outcome of each group were compared. The results showed that there were no significant differences in ovulation rate, pregnancy rate and live birth rate between the OCP pretreatment group and the control group. The ovulation rate, clinical pregnancy rate and live birth rate in the lifestyle intervention group were higher than those in the control group. The combined lifestyle and OCP intervention group had higher ovulation rate, clinical pregnancy rate and live birth rate than the control group, It was suggested that lifestyle adjustment or combined with OCP preconditioning could improve the success rate of clomiphene ovulation induction cycle.

However, some studies showed that lifestyle changes did not improve the outcome of assisted pregnancies in obese infertile women. In a randomized controlled study conducted by Mutsaerts et al. [31], the average weight of overweight/obese infertile patients decreased by 4.4 kg after 6 months of lifestyle intervention before assisted pregnancy treatment. However, the live birth rate in the intervention group was lower than that in the control group receiving direct assisted pregnancy treatment, and there was no significant difference between the pregnancy rate and the control group. van Oers et al. [32] further analyzed that there was no difference in the live birth rate between the obese and control group when assisted pregnancy treatment after 6 months of lifestyle preconditioning. Domecq et al. [33] conducted a meta-analysis on the pregnancy outcomes of PCOS patients with lifestyle intervention before assisting pregnancy and showed that there was no significant difference in clinical pregnancy rate between the lifestyle intervention group and the control group.

Up to 50–70% of PCOS patients were overweight or obese. Obesity, insulin resistance and secondary hyperinsulinemia were correlated with each other. Excessive insulin stimulated ovary to synthesize androgen and inhibit SHBG, which jointly led to the high androgen status in clinical manifestations and biochemical level of PCOS patients. Weight loss with adjusting lifestyle could improve central obesity, enhance insulin sensitivity, decrease fasting insulin and blood glucose levels, increase SHBG levels and reduce total and free testosterone levels, improve ovulation function and restore regular menstrual cycles [33–37].

Weight loss with adjusting lifestyle improved ovulation and intimal function. Ujvari et al. [38] analyzed for the first time the effects of weight reduction by lifestyle adjustment on intima gene expression and insulin signaling pathway in overweight/obese PCOS patients. The expression of endometrial insulin receptor substrate-1 (IRS-1) gene was significantly lower than that in the control group in proliferating phase of PCOS women. After overweight/obese PCOS patients received lifestyle intervention for 3 months, the average weight decreased by 4.7%, fasting insulin decreased significantly, menstruation returned to normal in 65% of subjects and 35% restored ovulation. Meanwhile, subjects of the intervention group had up-regulated mRNA levels of endometrial IRS-1 gene, which was positively correlated with increased mRNA levels of endometrial glucose transporter protein-1 (GLUT-1) gene. These results concluded that after the lifestyle intervention of obese PCOS patients, expression level of the insulin signaling pathway molecule in the endometrium was up-regulated to improve the endometrial function and promoted menstruation to return to normal.

Diet and exercise were beneficial to improve endocrine and metabolic functions. Jiskoot et al. [39] believed that multi-disciplinary lifestyle intervention through the combination of cognition, nutrition and exercise was more conducive to overweight/obese PCOS patients to develop a healthy lifestyle and achieved long-term weight loss, so as to improve the reproductive function, metabolic state and long-term life quality of overweight/obese PCOS women. A randomized controlled study of overweight/obese PCOS women followed a dietary intervention to lose weight for 4 months. The levels of anti-Müllerian hormone (AMH), total testosterone and free testosterone were significantly lower than those before intervention. Metabolic indicators including insulin growth factor (IGF-1) and insulin growth factor binding protein (IGFBP-1) were significantly higher than those before intervention, and insulin, blood sugar and insulin resistance index (HOMA-IR) were significantly lower than those before intervention [40]. Harrison et al. [15] reviewed the effects of exercise on PCOS patients and demonstrated that exercise therapy could improve ovulation function and insulin resistance and suggested that PCOS patients do moderate aerobic exercise for more than 90 min per week to improve reproductive and cardiovascular health. Dyslipidemia was a common cardiovascular risk factor in PCOS patients. Compared with moderate intensity exercise, PCOS subjects with high intensity exercise had higher levels of SHBG and high-density lipoprotein (HDL-C) and lower incidence of metabolic syndrome [41]. Other opinions held that lifestyle intervention had no significant improvement on dyslipidemia and OCP could improve HDL-C function, but lifestyle intervention combined with OCP drug therapy could improve HDL-C function and reduce the side effects of OCP on lipoprotein [42, 43]. Weight loss through diet and exercise intervention was important treatment strategies for PCOS patients, but studies have shown that the mechanisms of the two were different. Dietary intervention to reduce weight improved reproduction, psychology and metabolism of PCOS patients, which the mechanism may lie in the limitation of total energy intake. Palomba et al. [44] considered that after 24 weeks of exercise intervention, the weight loss of subjects was not as great as that of dietary intervention, but the ovulation rate was higher, which may be due to reduced insulin resistance and increased insulin sensitivity, thus improving the ovarian function. Therefore, dietary and exercise interventions for obese PCOS patients also need to be individualized.

Lifestyle intervention for weight loss regulated adipokine secretion. Fat cytokines synthesized and secreted by the fat tissues included adiponectin and leptin and inflammatory cytokines. Adiponectin was considered to be a preventive protective factor for obesity-related diseases such as diabetes and atherosclerosis, while leptin was a risk factor for cardiovascular disease. Obesity was often accompanied by characteristic high leptin levels and it is believed that obese people may exist leptin resistance [45, 46]. Adipocytokines were involved in regulating insulin sensitivity and affecting ovulation and fertilized egg planting. Adipocytokine secretion levels obese patients were changed, including decreased adiponectin levels, increased leptin and inflammatory of cytokines interleukin (IL)-6 and tumor necrosis factor (TNF-α) levels, which may be the possible mechanism of adverse pregnancy outcomes in obese women [21]. Adiponectin level was significantly correlated with visceral and subcutaneous fat. Subcutaneous and visceral fat decreased and adiponectin levels increased after weight loss by lifestyle intervention [22]. The prospective study of Siegrist et al. [23] showed that after 4–6 weeks of lifestyle intervention, the average weight of 402 obese subjects decreased by 8.9 kg, the serum adiponectin level increased, leptin and insulin levels decreased. Weight reduction with lifestyle intervention helped to regulate the secretion of adipokine. It may be one of the important mechanisms to improve PCOS dysfunction by weight loss.

3. Effects of exercise or combination with other methods on metabolic abnormalities in PCOS patients

PCOS was an endocrine disorder syndrome which coexists with reproductive dysfunction and metabolic abnormality. The clinical symptoms and long-term complications of PCOS patients were inseparable from their metabolic dysfunction. Studies have shown that excessive androgen and abnormal lipid metabolism were the main factors leading to skin characteristics (such as acne, hairy, male alopecia, etc.) in PCOS patients. The abdominal subcutaneous adipose tissue of obese PCOS patients was closely related to insulin resistance and androgen. Overweight could lead to lower levels of sex hormone binding globulin and increased androgen and insulin secretion and insulin resistance. This vicious circle would aggravate the clinical symptoms and signs of PCOS patients [47].

Brown et al. [48] showed that body composition (BMI, WHR and body fat rate) was significantly reduced after 12 weeks of aerobic exercise, and exercise and physical activity could reduce the storage of estrogen in body fat and promote the production of steroid hormones. Aerobic exercise significantly reduced the levels of SHBG and LH [49]. In the ovary, decreasing insulin levels reduced the level of androgen, WHR was the abdominal obesity index, and there was a relationship between WHR changes, body fat percentage and insulin sensitivity [50]. Therefore, reducing WHR and body fat percentage through aerobic exercise could increase the body's sensitivity to insulin and promote the production of SHBG. Androgen production was reduced and ovulation was promoted by increasing SHBG [49]. In the study conducted by Brown et al. [48], after 20 weeks of exercise, cholesterol, HDL and LDL levels were significantly improved. Regular endurance exercise could reduce TC, TG, LDL levels and increase HDL. PCOS patients had an increased risk of type 2 diabetes, dyslipidemia and cardiovascular disease. Moderate intensity exercise improved the composition of lipoprotein [51]. A prospective study by Salama et al. [28] convened 75 overweight/obese PCOS women and implemented a low-calorie diet and exercise intervention for 12 weeks. The average body weight of the subjects decreased by 6.3 kg, the body fat rate and visceral fat area decreased by 9.2 and 21.7% respectively, and the average blood pressure decreased from 124/82 mmHg to 120/80 mmHg, with statistically significant differences. In terms of metabolism, fasting blood glucose decreased by 5.15%, fasting insulin decreased by 27.86%, total cholesterol and triglyceride decreased by 8.9 and 18.02% respectively. In terms of endocrine metabolism, free testosterone index and SHBG decreased by 31 and 65.6% respectively. In addition, levels of inflammatory cytokines decreased after lifestyle intervention. Domecq et al. [33] conducted a meta-analysis on the pregnancy outcomes of PCOS patients with lifestyle intervention before assisting pregnancy and showed that weigh loss with adjusting lifestyle could reduce fasting insulin and fasting glucose, BMI decline was associated with reduced fasting blood glucose, these would help improve glucose metabolism. Based on previous research data, high-protein diet combined with regular exercise was adopted as the first-line treatment for obese PCOS patients and the results showed that after treatment, the patient's BMI was significantly reduced and the levels of LH, T, fasting blood glucose and insulin, IR and TG were decreased, but HDL was increased. Mehrabani et al. [52] demonstrated that the high-protein diet could significantly reduce the levels of BMI, T, insulin and IR. There were no significant changes in lipid and LH levels except LDL. Studies showed that after 8–12 weeks of moderate intensity exercise, the relevant indexes of lipid metabolism in PCOS patients could be significantly improved [48].

At present, modern medicine believed that the mechanism of exercise regulating metabolism may be related to the hormones involved in energy metabolism. Exercise could strengthen resting energy consumption (REE) of PCOS patients and reduce the content of adipose tissue in PCOS patients. REE of PCOS patients decreased compared with healthy women of the same age and BMI. Studies have shown that REE in obese people was significantly lower than that in non-obese one [53]. Therefore, REE may be declined in PCOS patients. Georgopoulos et al. [54] have also shown that there was a reduction of REE in PCOS patients, which be associated with increased fat content in the patients. On the other hand, exercise had a profound impact on the neuro-endocrine system, especially on the hormones involved in the regulation of energy metabolism, such as insulin, androgen, lactone and leptin. First, insulin resistance was the pathological basis of PCOS. It was generally agreed that one of the causes of insulin resistance was the abnormality of insulin signal pathway. Exercise or exercise training could affect the insulin action pathway from the three levels of pre-receptor, receptor and post-receptor in the pancreas islet [55]. Secondly, leptin played an important role in PCOS metabolism. Existing research showed that long-term exercise could reduce serum leptin level, improve leptin resistance and the sensitivity of the body to leptin. After sensitization, leptin could further inhibit the excessive secretion of insulin and the occurrence of hyperinsulinism, thus improve IR [56]. Thirdly, prolonged and intense exercise caused a decrease in blood testosterone, which may be caused by the body's hormones and some trace elements. For example, long time exercise or exercise training had obvious influence on zinc and selenium, zinc and selenium deficiency caused serum testosterone to drop [57]. Finally, some scholars have found that exercise could improve the expression of visfatin and promote the differentiation of visceral fat cells, and the differentiated fat cells contained a large number of insulin receptors, thus improving the sensitivity of insulin. Exercise may also promote necrosis and apoptosis of large adipocytes differentiated in visceral tissue, thereby reducing visceral adipocytes, improving insulin sensitivity and lipid metabolism disorder in the body [58].

4. The influence of exercise or combination with other methods on negative emotions of PCOS patients

In contemporary society, fierce competition, heavy work and study tasks, stay up late, lack of exercise and bad eating habits tended to cause stress reactions such as mental tension and emotional fluctuations in women which lead to endocrine imbalance in the hypothalamic-pituitary-ovarian gonadal axis, thus inducing PCOS. At the same time, PCOS patients were more likely to have severe inferiority complex, anxiety, depression and other abnormal psychological reactions than normal women [59]. It was reported that 17.19% patients with PCOS had anxiety, 32.81% had depression, and 10.15% had both depression and anxiety [60, 61]. Sudden or long-term mental depression, tension, anxiety, fear, depression, etc. could lead to mental endocrine disorders, menstrual and ovulation dysfunction, which aggravate the condition of PCOS patients and ultimately not conducive to the treatment of PCOS patients [62]. Therefore, it is increasingly important to treat PCOS patients' psychological diseases and relieve their psychological pressure.

Professor from the British nutrition foundation said doing more exercise could go a long way in boosting your self-esteem, improving your mood and coping with stress. It may even help you sleep and prevent depression. Studies have shown that exercise had obvious effect on the improvement of people's mental health level. Morgan suggested that intense exercise reduced anxiety which lasts for 2–5 h and regular exercise decreased anxiety and depression and boosted self-esteem [63]. Exercise could improve the state of mind, reduce the level of anxiety and have a therapeutic effect on anxiety. Regular exercise could effectively improve the psychological state of PCOS patients, ensure the effect of life intervention, and improve their quality of life [44]. Large, medium and small exercise loads could effectively improve the anxiety level of patients with severe generalized anxiety disorder, but large and medium exercise could more effectively improve the anxiety level of patients with mental anxiety [64]. Studies have found that a combination of physical activity and dietary intervention in PCOS patients could reduce depression and improve their life quality [65]. Teede et al. showed that PCOS patients lost 5–10% of body weight, their reproductive, metabolic and psychological characteristics were improved, and their sexual satisfaction and life quality were also increased [66].

For the regulation mechanism of negative emotions, exercise could increase the oxygen demand, improve the oxygen consumption and the cardiopulmonary function in human body. On the other hand, it could distract attention, transfer the experience of bad emotions, to achieve a comfortable body and mind and regulate emotions. Sports could produce a wealth of emotional experience and obtain more sports pleasure, comfort, satisfaction and fulfillment, showing an overall psychological state of good.

5. Conclusions

PCOS is a common reproductive endocrine disease in women of reproductive age. The clinical manifestations of PCOS patients are heterogeneous, it mainly affects reproductive, metabolic function and mental health. Its biochemical characteristics include insulin resistance, hyperinsulinemia, androgen overload and imbalance of LH/FSH ratio. Clinical manifestations include obesity, hirsute, acne and other high androgen symptoms, irregular ovulation or anovulation, menstrual disorders and infertility, bilateral polycystic changes of ovaries under ultrasound, and increased ovarian volume.

As one of the important treatment strategies for PCOS patients, adjusting lifestyle to lose weight was helpful to improve endocrine disorders and reduce the risk of metabolic syndrome, which is widely used in clinical practice. For obese PCOS patients who receive assisted pregnancy treatment, dietary and exercise intervention before assisted pregnancy could help restore spontaneous ovulation and enhance natural pregnancy rate, improve the outcome of assisted pregnancy, increase the success rate of assisted pregnancy and reduce the risk of pregnancy complications. Compared with weight-loss surgery, ovulatory drugs and IVF assisted pregnancy treatment, lifestyle adjustment for weight loss had unique advantages such as strong feasibility, low cost and large benefits. However, how to maintain reasonable, stable and long-term weight loss and keep target weight was still a big problem. In recent years, multidisciplinary cooperation involving diet, exercise and psychosocial intervention to guide obesity PCOS weight loss had attracted more and more attention, which is of great significance to guide clinicians to formulate more scientific and effective individual weight loss programs, improve the outcome of assisted pregnancy and long-term life quality of obese PCOS patients.

Acknowledgements

The study was supported by the Fujian Provincial Natural Science Foundation (2017 J01626 and 2017 J01627).

Conflict of interest

None.

Author details

Shaobing Wang*, Zhenghong Zhang and Yiping Liu
Provincial University Key Laboratory of Sport and Health Science, School of Physical Education and Sport Sciences, State Key Laboratory for Evaluation of Exercise Physiological Functions, General Administration of Sport of China, Fujian Normal University, Fuzhou, China

*Address all correspondence to: wshbingcn@fjnu.edu.cn

References

[1] Li R, Zhang Q, Yang D, Li S, Lu S, Wu X, et al. Prevalence of polycystic ovary syndrome in women in China: A large community-based study. Human Reproduction. 2013;**28**(9):2562-2569. DOI: 10.1093/humrep/det262

[2] Daan NM, Louwers YV, Koster MP, Eijkemans MJ, de Rijke YB, Lentjes EW, et al. Cardiovascular and metabolic profiles amongst different polycystic ovary syndrome phenotypes: Who is really at risk? Fertility and Sterility. 2014;**102**(5):1444-1451.e3. DOI: 10.1016/j.fertnstert.2014.08.001

[3] Mahalingaiah S, Diamanti-Kandarakis E. Targets to treat metabolic syndrome in polycystic ovary syndrome. Expert Opinion on Therapeutic Targets. 2015;**19**(11):1561-1574. DOI: 10.1517/14728222.2015.1101067

[4] Messinis IE, Messini CI, Anifandis G, Dafopoulos K. Polycystic ovaries and obesity. Best Practice & Research. Clinical Obstetrics & Gynaecology. 2015;**29**(4):479-488. DOI: 10.1016/j.bpobgyn.2014.11.001

[5] Cosar E, Uçok K, Akgün L, Köken G, Sahin FK, Arioz DT, et al. Body fat composition and distribution in women with polycystic ovary syndrome. Gynecological Endocrinology. 2008;**24**(8):428-432. DOI: 10.1080/09513590802234253

[6] Borruel S, Fernández-Durán E, Alpañés M, Martí D, Alvarez-Blasco F, Luque-Ramírez M, et al. Global adiposity and thickness of intraperitoneal and mesenteric adipose tissue depots are increased in women with polycystic ovary syndrome (PCOS). The Journal of Clinical Endocrinology and Metabolism. 2013;**98**(3):1254-1263. DOI: 10.1210/jc.2012-3698

[7] Motta AB. The role of obesity in the development of polycystic ovary syndrome. Current Pharmaceutical Design. 2012;**18**(17):2482-2491

[8] Lin AW, Lujan ME. Comparison of dietary intake and physical activity between women with and without polycystic ovary syndrome: A review. Advances in Nutrition. 2014;**5**(5):486-496

[9] Cui N, Wang H, Wang W, Zhang J, Xu Y, Jiang L, et al. Impact of body mass index on outcomes of In vitro fertilization/intracytoplasmic sperm injection among polycystic ovarian syndrome patients. Cellular Physiology and Biochemistry. 2016;**39**(5):1723-1734. DOI: 10.1159/000447873

[10] Koning AM, Kuchenbecker WK, Groen H, Hoek A, Land JA, Khan KS, et al. Economic consequences of overweight and obesity in infertility: A framework for evaluating the costs and outcomes of fertility care. Human Reproduction Update. 2010;**16**(3):246-254. DOI: 10.1093/humupd/dmp053

[11] Wang F, Dai W, Yang XH, Guo YH, Sun YP. Analyses of optimal body mass index for infertile patients with either polycystic or non-polycystic ovary syndrome during assisted reproductive treatment in China. Scientific Reports. 2016;**6**:34538. DOI: 10.1038/srep34538

[12] Stepto NK, Cassar S, Joham AE, Hutchison SK, Harrison CL, Goldstein RF, et al. Women with polycystic ovary syndrome have intrinsic insulin resistance on euglycaemic-hyperinsulaemic clamp. Human Reproduction. 2013;**28**(3):777-784. DOI: 10.1093/humrep/des463. Epub 2013 Jan 12

[13] Kyaw Tun T, McGowan A, Phelan N, Correia N, Boran G, O'Connor AL, et al. Obesity and insulin resistance are the main determinants of postprandial lipoprotein dysmetabolism in polycystic

ovary syndrome. International Journal of Endocrinology. 2016;**2016**:9545239. DOI: 10.1155/2016/9545239

[14] Rojas J, Chávez M, Olivar L, Rojas M, Morillo J, Mejías J, et al. Polycystic ovary syndrome, insulin resistance, and obesity: Navigating the pathophysiologic labyrinth. International Journal of Reproductive Medicine. 2014;**2014**:719050. DOI: 10.1155/2014/719050

[15] Harrison CL, Lombard CB, Moran LJ, Teede HJ. Exercise therapy in polycystic ovary syndrome: A systematic review. Human Reproduction Update. 2011;**17**(2):171-183. DOI: 10.1093/humupd/dmq045

[16] Palomba S, de Wilde MA, Falbo A, Koster MP, La Sala GB, Fauser BC. Pregnancy complications in women with polycystic ovary syndrome. Human Reproduction Update. 2015;**21**(5):575-592. DOI: 10.1093/humupd/dmv029

[17] Spritzer PM, Lecke SB, Satler F, Morsch DM. Adipose tissue dysfunction, adipokines, and low-grade chronic inflammation in polycystic ovary syndrome. Reproduction. 2015;**149**(5):R219-R227. DOI: 10.1530/REP-14-0435

[18] Heymsfield SB, Wadden TA. Mechanisms pathphysilogy and management of obesity. The New England Journal of Medicine. 2017;**376**:254-266

[19] Thomson RL, Buckley JD, Brinkworth GD. Exercise for the treatment and management of overweight women with polycystic ovary syndrome: A review of the literature. Obesity Reviews. 2011;**12**(5):e202-e210. DOI: 10.1111/j.1467-789X.2010.00758.x

[20] Tsagareli V, Noakes M, Norman RJ. Effect of a very-low-calorie diet on in vitro fertilization outcomes. Fertility and Sterility. 2006;**86**(1):227-229. DOI: 10.1016/j.fertnstert.2005.12.041

[21] Gosman GG, Katcher HI, Legro RS. Obesity and the role of gut and adipose hormones in female reproduction. Human Reproduction Update. 2006;**12**(5):585-601. DOI: 10.1093/humupd/dml024

[22] Zhang C, Luo H, Gao F, Zhang CT, Zhang R. A reduction in both visceral and subcutaneous fats contributes to increased adiponectin by lifestyle intervention in the Diabetes Prevention Program. Acta Diabetologica. 2015;**52**(3):625-628. DOI: 10.1007/s00592-014-0655-2

[23] Siegrist M, Rank M, Wolfarth B, Langhof H, Haller B, Koenig W, et al. Leptin, adiponectin, and short-term and long-term weight loss after a lifestyle intervention in obese children. Nutrition. 2013;**29**(6):851-857. DOI: 10.1016/j.nut.2012.12.011. Epub 2013 Feb 16

[24] Hollmann M, Runnebaum B, Gerhard I. Effects of weight loss on the hormonal profile in obese, infertile women. Human Reproduction. 1996;**11**(9):1884-1891. DOI: 10.1093/oxfordjournals.humrep.a019512

[25] Hoeger KM. Role of lifestyle modification in the management of polycystic ovary syndrome. Best Practice & Research. Clinical Endocrinology & Metabolism. 2006;**20**(2):293-310. DOI: 10.1016/j.beem.2006.03.008

[26] Huber-Buchholz MM, Carey DG, Norman RJ. Restoration of reproductive potential by lifestyle modification in obese polycystic ovary syndrome: Role of insulin sensitivity and luteinizing hormone. The Journal of Clinical Endocrinology and Metabolism. 1999;**84**(4):1470-1474. DOI: 10.1210/jcem.84.4.5596

[27] Kuchenbecker WK, Groen H, van Asselt SJ, Bolster JH, Zwerver J, Slart RH, et al. In women with polycystic ovary syndrome and obesity, loss of intra-abdominal fat is associated with resumption of ovulation. Human Reproduction. 2011;**26**(9):2505-2512. DOI: 10.1093/humrep/der229

[28] Salama AA, Amine EK, Salem HA, Abd El Fattah NK. Anti-inflammatory dietary combo in overweight and obese women with polycystic ovary syndrome. North American Journal of Medical Sciences. 2015;**7**(7):310-316. DOI: 10.4103/1947-2714.161246

[29] Legro RS, Dodson WC, Kris-Etherton PM, Kunselman AR, Stetter CM, Williams NI, et al. Randomized controlled trial of preconception interventions in infertile women with polycystic ovary syndrome. The Journal of Clinical Endocrinology and Metabolism. 2015;**100**(11):4048-4058. DOI: 10.1210/jc.2015-2778

[30] Legro RS, Dodson WC, Kunselman AR, Stetter CM, Kris-Etherton PM, Williams NI, et al. Benefit of delayed fertility therapy with preconception weight loss over immediate therapy in obese women with PCOS. The Journal of Clinical Endocrinology and Metabolism. 2016;**101**(7):2658-2666. DOI: 10.1210/jc.2016-1659

[31] Mutsaerts MA, van Oers AM, Groen H, Burggraaff JM, Kuchenbecker WK, Perquin DA, et al. Randomized trial of a lifestyle program in obese infertile women. The New England Journal of Medicine. 2016;**374**(20):1942-1953. DOI: 10.1056/NEJMoa1505297

[32] van Oers AM, Groen H, Mutsaerts MA, Burggraaff JM, Kuchenbecker WK, Perquin DA, et al., LIFEstyle study group. Effectiveness of lifestyle intervention in subgroups of obese infertile women: A subgroup analysis of a RCT. Human Reproduction. 2016;**31**(12):2704-2713. DOI: 10.1093/humrep/dew252

[33] Domecq JP, Prutsky G, Mullan RJ, Hazem A, Sundaresh V, Elamin MB, et al. Lifestyle modification programs in polycystic ovary syndrome: Systematic review and meta-analysis. The Journal of Clinical Endocrinology and Metabolism. 2013;**98**(12):4655-4663. DOI: 10.1210/jc.2013-2385

[34] Tannus S, Burke YZ, Kol S. Treatment strategies for the infertile polycystic ovary syndrome patient. Women's Health (London, England). 2015;**11**(6):901-912. DOI: 10.2217/whe.15.40

[35] Moran LJ, Hutchison SK, Norman RJ, Teede HJ. Lifestyle changes in women with polycystic ovary syndrome. Cochrane Database of Systematic Reviews. 2011;7:CD007506. DOI: 10.1002/14651858.CD007506.pub3

[36] Mahoney D. Lifestyle modification intervention among infertile overweight and obese women with polycystic ovary syndrome. Journal of the American Association of Nurse Practitioners. 2014;**26**(6):301-308. DOI: 10.1002/2327-6924.12073

[37] Phy JL, Pohlmeier AM, Cooper JA, Watkins P, Spallholz J, Harris KS, et al. Low starch/low dairy diet results in successful treatment of obesity and co-morbidities linked to polycystic ovary syndrome (PCOS). Journal of Obesity and Weight Loss Therapy. 2015;**5**(2). pii: 259. DOI: 10.4172/2165-7904.1000259

[38] Ujvari D, Hulchiy M, Calaby A, Nybacka Å, Byström B, Hirschberg AL. Lifestyle intervention up-regulates gene and protein levels of molecules involved in insulin signaling in the endometrium of overweight/obese women with polycystic ovary

syndrome. Human Reproduction. 2014;**29**(7):1526-1535

[39] Jiskoot G, Benneheij SH, Beerthuizen A, de Niet JE, de Klerk C, Timman R, et al. A three-component cognitive behavioural lifestyle program for preconceptional weight-loss in women with polycystic ovary syndrome (PCOS): A protocol for a randomized controlled trial. Reproductive Health. 2017;**14**(1):34. DOI: 10.1186/s12978-017-0295-4

[40] Nybacka Å, Carlström K, Fabri F, Hellström PM, Hirschberg AL. Serum antimüllerian hormone in response to dietary management and/or physical exercise in overweight/obese women with polycystic ovary syndrome: Secondary analysis of a randomized controlled trial. Fertility and Sterility. 2013;**100**(4):1096-1102. DOI: 10.1016/j.fertnstert.2013.06.030

[41] Greenwood EA, Noel MW, Kao CN, Shinkai K, Pasch LA, Cedars MI, et al. Vigorous exercise is associated with superior metabolic profiles in polycystic ovary syndrome independent of total exercise expenditure. Fertility and Sterility. 2016;**105**(2):486-493. DOI: 10.1016/j.fertnstert.2015.10.020

[42] Macut D, Bjekić-Macut J, Savić-Radojević A. Dyslipidemia and oxidative stress in PCOS. Frontiers of Hormone Research. 2013;**40**:51-63. DOI: 10.1159/000341683

[43] Dokras A, Playford M, Kris-Etherton PM, Kunselman AR, Stetter CM, Williams NI, et al. Impact of hormonal contraception and weight loss on high-density lipoprotein cholesterol efflux and lipoprotein particles in women with polycystic ovary syndrome. Clinical Endocrinology. 2017;**86**(5): 739-746. DOI: 10.1111/cen.13310

[44] Palomba S, Giallauria F, Falbo A, Russo T, Oppedisano R, Tolino A, et al. Structured exercise training programme versus hypocaloric hyperproteic diet in obese polycystic ovary syndrome patients with anovulatory infertility: A 24-week pilot study. Human Reproduction. 2008;**23**(3):642-650. DOI: 10.1093/humrep/dem391

[45] Smekal A, Vaclavik J. Adipokines and cardiovascular disease: A comprehensive review. Biomedical Papers of the Medical Faculty of the University Palacky, Olomouc, Czech Republic. 2017;**161**(1):31-40. DOI: 10.5507/bp.2017.002

[46] López-Jaramillo P, Gómez-Arbeláez D, López-López J, López-López C, Martínez-Ortega J, Gómez-Rodríguez A, et al. The role of leptin/adiponectin ratio in metabolic syndrome and diabetes. Hormone Molecular Biology and Clinical Investigation. 2014;**18**(1):37-45. DOI: 10.1515/hmbci-2013-0053

[47] Wehr E, Möller R, Horejsi R, Giuliani A, Kopera D, Schweighofer N, et al. Subcutaneous adipose tissue topography and metabolic disturbances in polycystic ovary syndrome. Wiener Klinische Wochenschrift. 2009;**121**(7-8):262-269. DOI: 10.1007/s00508-009-1162-2

[48] Brown AJ, Setji TL, Sanders LL, Lowry KP, Otvos JD, Kraus WE, et al. Effects of exercise on lipoprotein particles in women with polycystic ovary syndrome. Medicine and Science in Sports and Exercise. 2009;**41**(3):497-504. DOI: 10.1249/MSS.0b013e31818c6c0c

[49] Lord JM, Flight IH, Norman RJ. Metformin in polycystic ovary syndrome: Systematic review and meta-analysis. BMJ. 2003;**327**(7421):951-953. DOI: 10.1136/bmj.327.7421.951

[50] Tymchuk CN, Tessler SB, Barnard RJ. Changes in sex hormone-binding globulin, insulin, and serum

lipids in postmenopausal women on a low-fat, high-fiber diet combined with exercise. Nutrition and Cancer. 2000;**38**(2):158-162. DOI: 10.1207/S15327914NC382_3

[51] Chan JL, Kar S, Vanky E, Morin-Papunen L, Piltonen T, Puurunen J, et al. Racial and ethnic differences in the prevalence of metabolic syndrome and its components of metabolic syndrome in women with polycystic ovary syndrome: A regional cross-sectional study. American Journal of Obstetrics and Gynecology. 2017;**217**(2):189.e1-189.e8. DOI: 10.1016/j.ajog.2017.04.007

[52] Mehrabani HH, Salehpour S, Amiri Z, Farahani SJ, Meyer BJ, Tahbaz F. Beneficial effects of a high-protein, low-glycemic-load hypocaloric diet in overweight and obese women with polycystic ovary syndrome: A randomized controlled intervention study. Journal of the American College of Nutrition. 2012;**31**(2):117-125

[53] Jia WP, Yang M, Shao XY, Bao YQ, Lu JX, Xiang KS. Resting energy expenditure and its relationship with patterns of obesity and visceral fat area in Chinese adults. Biomedical and Environmental Sciences. 2005;**18**(2):103-107

[54] Georgopoulos NA, Saltamavros AD, Vervita V, Karkoulias K, Adonakis G, Decavalas G, et al. Basal metabolic rate is decreased in women with polycystic ovary syndrome and biochemical hyperandrogenemia and is associated with insulin resistance. Fertility and Sterility. 2009;**92**(1):250-255. DOI: 10.1016/j.fertnstert.2008.04.067

[55] Moghetti P. Insulin resistance and polycystic ovary syndrome. Current Pharmaceutical Design. 2016;**22**(36):5526-5534

[56] Pehlivanov B, Mitkov M. Serum leptin levels correlate with clinical and biochemical indices of insulin resistance in women with polycystic ovary syndrome. The European Journal of Contraception & Reproductive Health Care. 2009;**14**(2):153-159. DOI: 10.1080/13625180802549962

[57] Shafiei Neek L, Gaeini AA, Choobineh S. Effect of zinc and selenium supplementation on serum testosterone and plasma lactate in cyclist after an exhaustive exercise bout. Biological Trace Element Research. 2011;**144**(1-3):454-462. DOI: 10.1007/s12011-011-9138-2

[58] Qi X, Zhang B, Zhao Y, Li R, Chang HM, Pang Y, et al. Hyperhomocysteinemia promotes insulin resistance and adipose tissue inflammation in PCOS mice through modulating M2 macrophage polarization via estrogen suppression. Endocrinology. 2017;**158**(5):1181-1193. DOI: 10.1210/en.2017-00039

[59] Coffey S, Bano G, Mason HD. Health-related quality of life in women with polycystic ovary syndrome: A comparison with the general population using the polycystic ovary syndrome questionnaire (PCOSQ) and the short Form-36 (SF-36). Gynecological Endocrinology. 2006;**22**(2):80-86. DOI: 10.1080/09513590600604541

[60] Bhattacharya SM, Jha A. Prevalence and risk of depressive disorders in women with polycystic ovary syndrome (PCOS). Fertility and Sterility. 2010;**94**(1):357-359. DOI: 10.1016/j.fertnstert.2009.09.025

[61] Deeks AA, Gibson-Helm ME, Teede HJ. Anxiety and depression in polycystic ovary syndrome: A comprehensive investigation. Fertility and Sterility. 2010;**93**(7):2421-2423. DOI: 10.1016/j.fertnstert.2009.09.018

[62] Bazarganipour F, Ziaei S, Montazeri A, Foroozanfard F, Kazemnejad A, Faghihzadeh S.Psycho-

logical investigation in patients with polycystic ovary syndrome. Health and Quality of Life Outcomes. 2013;**11**:141. DOI: 10.1186/1477-7525-11-141

[63] Morgan WP. Affective beneficence of vigorous physical activity. Medicine and Science in Sports and Exercise. 1985;**17**(1):94-100

[64] Conte F, Banting L, Teede HJ, Stepto NK. Mental health and physical activity in women with polycystic ovary syndrome: A brief review. Sports Medicine. 2015;**45**(4):497-504. DOI: 10.1007/s40279-014-0291-6

[65] Thomson RL, Buckley JD, Lim SS, Noakes M, Clifton PM, Norman RJ, et al. Lifestyle management improves quality of life and depression in overweight and obese women with polycystic ovary syndrome. Fertility and Sterility. 2010;**94**(5):1812-1816. DOI: 10.1016/j.fertnstert.2009.11.001

[66] Teede H, Deeks A, Moran L. Polycystic ovary syndrome: A complex condition with psychological, reproductive and metabolic manifestations that impacts on health across the lifespan. BMC Medicine. 2010;**8**:41. DOI: 10.1186/1741-7015-8-41

Chapter 4

Effect of Aromatase Inhibitors versus Clomiphene Citrate for Ovulation Induction in Infertile Women with Ovulatory Dysfunction (PCO)

Hassan S.O. Abduljabbar, Magda Hagras and Rania Magadmy

Abstract

A RCT conducted to assess the efficacy of letrozole as an ovulation induction agent in infertile women, and to compare the effectiveness of letrozole with the current standard agent, clomiphene citrate given for three successive cycles on the induction of ovulation. Forty-five infertile women with anovulation included, the subjects were randomly divided into two groups; subjects were allocated to either CC (100) or letrozole (5 mg) daily—5 days starting on the third day of menses, for 3 months. On stimulation day 12 subjects, serum estradiol and transvaginal sonography to document the number of follicles was done. On stimulation day 21 subjects, serum progesterone and ultrasound for the thickness of endometrium was done. Participants were followed up monthly. Results revealed that the mean number of follicles reaching >18 mm and endometrial thickness in the letrozole comparable to those receiving clomiphene citrate. Letrozole showed lower estradiol level compared to Clomiphene citrate ($P < 0.05$). Ovulation occurred in 84.4%, 78.1% in the letrozole and clomiphene citrate, respectively, and pregnancy rate is 18.8% in the letrozole group compared to 15% in the clomiphene citrate group. In conclusion, there was no significant increase in the number of follicles, endometrial thickness and pregnancy rate induced by letrozole compared with clomiphene citrate.

Keywords: infertility, anovulation, letrozole, clomiphene citrate

1. Introduction

Many controversies surround the treatment of infertile women with polycystic ovary syndrome (PCOS). Before any intervention is initiated, pre-conceptional counselling should be provided emphasizing the importance of lifestyle, especially weight reduction and exercise in overweight women, smoking, and alcohol consumption [1].

The recommended first-line treatment for ovulation induction remains the antiestrogen clomiphene citrate (CC). Recommended second-line intervention, should CC fail to result in pregnancy, is either exogenous gonadotropins or laparoscopic ovarian surgery (LOS). The use of exogenous gonadotropins is associated with increased chances for multiple pregnancies, and, therefore, intense monitoring of ovarian response is required. Laparoscopic ovarian surgery alone is usually effective in less than 50% of women, and additional ovulation induction medication is required under those circumstances. Recommended third-line treatment is in vitro fertilization (IVF) [1].

Aromatase inhibitors aromatase inhibitors act not only by decreasing circulating levels of estrogen, but also by directly blocking local estrogen production in the breast tumor.

In premenopausal women, it causes an increase in gonadotropin secretion because of the reduced negative feedback of estrogen to the pituitary.

It also leads to ovarian stimulation, an increase in ovarian size, which may result in ovarian cysts in premenopausal females [2].

Kafy and Tulandi [3] found that letrozole in a dose of 5 mg daily for 5 days is associated with a thicker endometrium and a better pregnancy rate. It is as effective as gonadotropin but yet less expensive. Moreover, induction of ovulation with FSH injections is carried with relative risks of multiple gestations and severe ovarian hyperstimulation syndrome [4]. The benefit of the use of aromatase inhibitors has not yet been proven in large studies [5].

Gregoriou et al. [6] stated that ovarian stimulation with letrozole is associated with acceptable pregnancy rates compared with gonadotropin with significant less cost, risks, and patient inconvenience. In addition, suggests that clomiphene suppresses endometrial receptivity more than letrozole, and they concluded that letrozole might be an appropriate drug for ovulation induction. Fortunately, Badawy et al. [7] documented safety of letrozole and clomiphene citrate for both the mother and fetuses.

Yet, the benefit of the use of aromatase inhibitors has not yet been proven in large studies, and further randomized-controlled studies are warranted to define more clearly the efficacy and safety of letrozole in human reproduction.

2. Material and methods

Condition phase: Infertility due to anovulation.

Intervention: Patients were assigned to the letrozole or clomiphene citrate. Patients were enrolled and followed-up. The Ethics Committee of the King Abdulaziz University Hospital approved this study. Written informed consent was obtained from each patient.

Study design: Treatment, randomized, double-blind, efficacy study comparing letrozole versus clomifene citrate for ovulation induction.

Setting: A university teaching hospital.

Primary outcome measures: Ovulation rate, number of growing and mature follicles during treatment, serum estradiol level, serum progesterone level, endometrial thickness.

Secondary outcome measures: Hyperstimulation, miscarriage rate, multiple pregnancy rate, and ectopic pregnancy trial population: 44 infertile females were assigned to the study according to certain inclusion criteria.

Inclusion criteria

1. Age: 25–40, BMI < 30.

2. Infertility due to anovulation.

3. No recent (within 3 months) treatment for induction of ovulation.

4. Normal semen analysis.

5. Proven patency of at least one fallopian tube.

6. Had no other pelvic pathology.

Exclusion criteria

1. Inability to give informed consent

2. Hypersensivity to letrozole or clomiphene citrate

3. Excess prolactin levels

4. Other causes of infertility

5. Absence of any inclusion criteria.

This double-blind randomized-controlled trial was conducted in 44 infertile patients attending the Department of Obstetrics and Gynecology, King Abdulaziz University Hospital, Jeddah over a period of 1 year. Forty-four infertile women, aged between 25 and 40 years with infertility for 2 years or more, of unprotected coitus without conception in patients who have never conceived before, because of anovulation related to PCOS, were recruited for study after obtaining informed consents from the couples. PCOS diagnosis required the presence of two of three criteria, i.e., oligomenorrhea and/or anovulation, clinical and biochemical signs of hyperandrogenism, and/or polycystic ovaries on ultrasound. Couples with any other significant subfertility factor in either of the partner detected by pre-recruitment investigations were not included in this study. The Ethics Committee of the King Abdulaziz University Hospital approved this study.

All patients were screened for the hormonal profile, including the follicle-stimulating hormone, luteinizing hormone, prolactin, thyroid-stimulating hormone, estradiol, a pelvic ultrasound for confirmation of polycystic changes in the ovary, hysterosalpingography to determine tubal patency, Semen analysis in the patient's partner to rule out malefactor.

Computer-assisted randomization was done and concealment was ensured. The candidates were randomly divided into two groups. Patients were allocated to either group (I), where patients received 5 mg of letrozole once daily (Femara®, Novartis, Basel, Switzerland), or group (II), where patients received 100 mg of CC once daily (Clomid®, Sanofi Aventis, France), for 5 days starting on day 3 of menses, for the first, second, and third month. Follow-up of ovulation and endometrial thickness was monitored by transvaginal ultrasonographic folliculometry by the same operator by the same observer. Timed intercourse was advised 24 h after measuring dominant follicle of >18 mm till 12 h post ovulation.

Subjects returned to the clinic on stimulation day 12 for blood sampling to analyze estradiol and were undergone transvaginal sonography to document on the number of follicles (Note: Stimulation day 1 equals the first day of study drug).

Blood sampling was repeated on stimulation day 21 for the analysis of serum progesterone. Ovulation was confirmed by a progesterone level 10 ng/mL. If the results of the progesterone test indicate that the patient has not ovulated, the subject was brought back 1–2 days later for a repeat progesterone test. Also, ultrasound for assessment of the thickness of the endometrium was done.

In ovulatory cycles, a pregnancy test was performed 3 days post missed period. Subjects with a positive pregnancy test were supplemented with micronized progesterone vaginally. Participants were evaluated for three courses of intervention.

Subjects may be allowed to continue for up to two additional treatment cycles if they failed to achieve clinical pregnancy in their first treatment cycle, and did not experience other mandatory withdrawal condition. A follow-up visit was arranged for each group every month at the second day of menstruation until 3 months after recruitment or at any time during the trial if the pregnancy was achieved.

2.1 Statistical analysis

The data were analyzed with the Statistical Program SPSS version 16. Descriptive statistics comprised the mean and standard deviation (SD), analytical statistics comprised the t-test to make comparisons between independent quantitative means, and the Anova test to make comparisons between the different groups. P value < 0.05 was significant. Pearson correlation was done between different parameters.

3. Results

Results obtained during the term of the project and data analysis. Patients were randomized so as, 24 women of mean age (30.2 ± 4.3) years received letrozole; whereas, 20 women of mean age (29.8 ± 4.7) years received clomiphene citrate. Group (I) had a body mass index of (28.2 ± 2.1); whereas, group (II) had a body mass index of (27.4 ± 2.2). There was no significant difference between the groups as regard age or body mass index (P > 0.05) (**Table 1**) and the baseline hormonal profiles of the two groups (**Table 2**).

There was no significant statistical difference between letrozole group and the clomiphene citrate group concerning the following hormones: serum FSH day 2 (5.5 ± 1.9 versus 5.9 ± 1.5 IU/ml), serum LH day 2 (4.1 ± 2.4 versus 4.4 ± 2.3 mIU/ml), and serum E2 day 2 (53.1 ± 11.4 versus 50.9 ± 15 pmol/L).

	Age	**BMI**
Letrozole (n = 24)	30.2 ± 4.3	28.2 ± 2.1
Clomiphene citrate (n = 20)	29.8 ± 4.7	27.4 ± 2.2
Significance	NS	NS

Significant change: P < 0.05.

Table 1.
Baseline parameters of the study groups.

	FSH	**LH**	**TSH**	**Prolactin**	**Estradiol**
	IU/ml	**mlU/ml**	**ulU/m**	**mlU/L**	**pmol/L**
Letrozole (n = 24)	5.5 ± 1.9	4.1 ± 2.4	1.9 ± 0.1	12.2 ± 2.6	53.1 ± 11.4
Clomiphene citrate (n = 20)	5.9 ± 1.5	4.4 ± 2.3	2.0 ± 0.2	13.4 ± 1.6	50.9 ± 15
Significance	NS	NS	NS	NS	NS

Significant change: P < 0.05.

Table 2.
Baseline hormonal parameters of the study groups.

The primary outcome measures were a number of mature follicles and endometrial thickness (in mm); secondary outcome measures were the pregnancy rate and miscarriage rate. The number of follicles showed no statistically significant ($P > 0.05$) difference between the groups (5.8 ± 3.6 for Group I versus 3.2 ± 3.3 in Group II) in cycle I. Endometrial thickness showed no statistically significant ($P > 0.05$) difference (9.07 ± 0.3 for Group I versus 4.08 ± 0.3 cm for Group II) (**Table 3**).

The mean number of follicles reaching >18 mm was significantly higher in patients who received letrozole (4.5 ± 4.5) than in those receiving clomiphene citrate (3.6 ± 3.6), although this difference was found non-significant. Letrozole and clomiphene citrate showing no significant difference ($P > 0.05$) as regards the endometrial thickness (1.1 ± 0.2 versus 1.2 ± 0.2) (**Table 3**). There is an insignificant difference between clomiphene citrate and letrozole as regard endometrial thickness and number of follicles through the 3 cycles. Clomiphene citrate significantly increased estradiol and progesterone levels compared to letrozole in cycle 1 and cycle 3 (**Tables 3–5**).

	Estradiol	Progesterone	Follicles	Endometrium	Pregnancy
	pmol/L	mol/L	Number	Thickness (cm)	Rate
Letrozole (n = 24)	4.5 ± 455.7*	47.6 ± 34.4	4.5 ± 4.5	1.1.2 ± 0.2	2.0
CC (n = 20)	2.5 ± 2127.6	62.2 ± 62.8	3.6 ± 3.6	1.2 ± 0.2	1.9 ± 0.2
Significance	0.001	0.017	0.820	0.724	0.030

CC = clomiphene citrate.
Significant change: P < 0.05.

Table 3.
Effect of letrozole versus clomiphene citrate on estradiol, progesterone, no. of follicles and endometrial thickness in cycle 1.

	Estradiol	Progesterone	Follicles	Endometrium	Pregnancy
	pmol/L	mol/L	Number	Thickness (cm)	Rate
Letrozole (n = 24)	4.2 ± 656.7*	39.6 ± 31.1	5.8 ± 3.6*	1.07 ± 0.3	1.8 ± 0.3
CC (n = 20)	1.5 ± 904.5	48.9 ± 57.1	3.2 ± 3.3	1.08 ± .3	2.0 ± 0.2
Significance	0.25	0.14	0.46	0.81	0.02

CC = clomiphene citrate.
Significant change: P < 0.05.

Table 4.
Effect of letrozole versus clomiphene citrate on estradiol, progesterone, no. of follicles and endometrial thickness in cycle 2.

	Estradiol	Progesterone	Follicles	Endometrium	Pregnancy
	pmol/L	mol/L	Number	Thickness (cm)	Rate
Letrozole (n = 24)	3.9 ± 349.09	36.8 ± 26	5.1 ± 4.8	1.05 ± 0.2	2.0 ± 0.3
CC (n = 20)	4.08 ± 5443.4	51.3 ± 68.5	1.3 ± 1.5	1.09 ± 0.4	2.0 ± 0.2
Significance	0.007	0.05	0.26	0.10	NS

CC = clomiphene citrate.
Significant change: P < 0.05.

Table 5.
Effect of Letrozole versus clomiphene citrate on estradiol, progesterone, no. of follicles and endometrial thickness in cycle 3.

	No. of pregnancy	Miscarriage
Letrozole (n = 24)	4	0
Clomiphene citrate (n = 20)	3	0
Significance	0.49	NS

Significant change: P < 0.05.

Table 6.
Effect of letrozole versus clomiphene citrate on number of pregnancies pregnancy and miscarriages in the 3 cycles.

A comparison of the number of pregnancies achieved in the groups showed insignificant statistical difference ($P < 0.05$). No multiple pregnancies occurred in both groups (**Table 6**).

Anova between the 3 cycles revealed that there is no significant difference between estradiol, progesterone levels, number of follicles, and endometrial thickness. Post Hoc Tests also revealed insignificant differences between the outcomes in the 3 cycles.

4. Discussion

Detailed scientific discussions of the results obtained during the term of the project, and related past results obtained in the field of this research area. Although clomiphene citrate is considered the first-line drug for ovulation induction in women with PCOS, a significant proportion of women do not respond to this treatment [8]. Letrozole, a third-generation aromatase inhibitor, is suggested for ovulation induction [9].

Letrozole initiates ovulation by decreasing the conversion of androstenedione and testosterone to estrogen in the ovary. The inhibition of estrogen production, in turn, increases GnRH release and pituitary follicle-stimulating hormone (FSH) synthesis [10]. Clomiphene citrate acts by blocking the negative feedback of endogenous estrogen at the level of the hypothalamus and pituitary gland and promoting an increase in the pulsatile release of luteinizing hormone and follicle-stimulating hormone. However, clomiphene citrate has an antagonistic effect on the endometrium and may reduce endometrial thickness [11].

The results of this prospective randomized study showed that letrozole was as effective as clomiphene citrate for induction of ovulation with an insignificant change in the number of mature follicles and endometrial thickness. Atay et al. [8] reported that letrozole and clomiphene citrate were effective for ovulation induction in PCOS, but in contrast to the present study, they found greater endometrial thickness in the letrozole group.

In the present study, clomiphene citrate significantly increased estradiol and progesterone levels compared to letrozole in cycle one and cycle 3. Badawy et al. [7] found that levels of serum estradiol and progesterone were statistically significantly higher in the clomiphene citrate group compared to letrozole.

The hormonal changes could be explained by clomiphene citrate (CC) binds to estrogen receptors (ERs) for an extended period of time due to its structural similarity to estrogen. This will deplete ER concentrations. The antiestrogenic effect on the hypothalamus and the pituitary is believed to be the main mechanism of action for ovarian stimulation. Depletion of hypothalamic ERs prevents correct interpretation of circulating estrogen levels; estrogen concentrations are falsely perceived as low leading to reduced estrogen-negative feedback on GnRH production and subsequent increased gonadotropin (FSH and LH) secretion. The rise of FSH promotes growth of ovarian follicles and ovulation in anovulatory women. It is believed that the hypothalamus is the main site of action because in normally ovulatory women, CC treatment was found to increase GnRH pulse frequency [12].

Letrozole block estrogen-negative feedback, without depletion of ERs as occurs with CC. Inhibition of aromatization will block estrogen production from all sources and release the hypothalamic/pituitary axis from estrogenic negative feedback. The resultant increase in gonadotropin secretion will stimulate growth of ovarian follicles [13].

5. Conclusions and recommendations

Letrozole in patients with PCOS is as effective as clomiphene citrate in inducing ovulation; letrozole had a comparable effect to clomiphene citrate on endometrial thickness and number of follicles.

Acknowledgements

We thank Amani Al-Mars, Laila Al-Tonesy, Hala Al-Tayeb, and Amina Saleh for their contribution in collecting data.

Conflicts of interest

The authors of this paper report no conflicts of interest.

Author details

Hassan S.O. Abduljabbar[1*], Magda Hagras[1,2] and Rania Magadmy[3]

1 Faculty of Medicine, King Abdulaziz University, Kingdom of Saudi Arabia

2 Faculty of Medicine, Suez Canal University, Egypt

3 Clinical Trial Unit, King Fahd Medical Research Centre, King Abdulaziz University, Kingdom of Saudi Arabia

*Address all correspondence to: profaj17@yahoo.com

References

[1] Thessaloniki ESHRE/ASRM-Sponsored PCOS Consensus Workshop Group. Consensus on infertility treatment related to polycystic ovary syndrome. Human Reproduction. 2008;**23**(3):462-477. DOI: 10.1093/humrep/dem426. Erratum in: Hum Reprod. 2008;**23**(6):1474. PMID: 18308833

[2] Jermy K, Luise C, Bourne T. The characterization of common ovarian cysts in premenopausal women. Ultrasound in Obstetrics and Gynecology. 2001;**17**(2):140-144

[3] Kafy S, Tulandi T. New advances in ovulation induction. Current Opinion in Obstetrics and Gynecology. 2007;**19**(3):248-252

[4] Nader S. Ovulation induction in polycystic ovary syndrome. Minerva Ginecologica. 2008;**60**(1):53-61. Review

[5] Hart R. PCOS and infertility. Panminerva Medica. 2008;**50**(4):305-314. Review

[6] Gregoriou MD, Nikos F, Vlahos MD. Randomized controlled trial comparing superovulation with letrozole versus recombinant follicle-stimulating hormone combined with intrauterine insemination for couples with unexplained infertility who had failed clomiphene citrate stimulation and intrauterine insemination. Fertility and Sterility. 2008;**90**(3):678-683. DOI: 10.1016/j.fertnstert.2007.06.099

[7] Badawy A, Shokeir T, Allam AF, Abdelhady H. Pregnancy outcome after ovulation induction with aromatase inhibitors or clomiphene citrate in unexplained infertility. Acta Obstetricia et Gynecologica Scandinavica. 2009;**88**(2):187-191. DOI: 10.1080/00016340802638199

[8] Atay V, Cam C, Muhcu M, Cam M, Karateke A. Comparison of letrozole and clomiphene citrate in women with polycystic ovaries undergoing ovarian stimulation. The Journal of International Medical Research. 2006;**34**(1):73-76

[9] Ekerhovd E. Ovulation induction by means of letrozole. Tidsskrift for den Norske Lægeforening. 2009;**129**(5):412-415. DOI: 10.4045/tidsskr.08.0129. Review. Norwegian

[10] Ohno Y, Fujimoto Y. Endometrial oestrogen and progesterone receptors and their relationship to sonographic appearance of the endometrium. Human Reproduction Update. 1998;**4**(5):560-564. Review

[11] Nakamura Y, Ono M, Yoshida Y, Sugino N, Ueda K, Kato H. Effects of clomiphene citrate on the endometrial thickness and echogenic pattern of the endometrium. Fertility and Sterility. 1997;**67**(2):256-260

[12] Kerin JF, Liu JH, Phillipou G, Yen SS. Evidence for a hypothalamic site of action of clomiphene citrate in women. The Journal of Clinical Endocrinology and Metabolism. 1985;**61**(2):265-268

[13] Kamath MS, George K. Letrozole or clomiphene citrate as first line for anovulatory infertility: A debate. Reproductive Biology and Endocrinology. 2011;**9**:86. DOI: 10.1186/1477-7827-9-86

Section 2

Basic Researches of Polycystic Ovary Syndrome

Chapter 5

Endocrine Characteristics and Regulatory Mechanism of Follicular Development and Ovulation Failure in Mammalian Ovary

Zhenghong Zhang, Yan Zhang, Fengping Lin and Zhengchao Wang

Abstract

In mammals, the follicular development and following ovulation are regulated by reproductive hormones, while polycystic ovary syndrome (PCOS) is an endocrine disorder syndrome with reproductive dysfunction and abnormal glucose metabolism in most PCOS women. Its characteristics are hyperandrogenism, ovarian dysfunction, and the exclusion of other androgen excess or related diseases. Its clinical characteristics are large antral follicle pool from which to recruit and persistent anovulation. The incidence of PCOS in women of childbearing age ranged from 4 to 12%. About one-third of infertility cases had no ovulation, and 90% of them had PCOS. Therefore, further studying the regulatory mechanism of follicular hyperrecruitment and anovulation can provide theoretical basis for exploring the pathogenesis of PCOS and guiding clinical treatment, especially for protecting female fertility and preventing the occurrence of metabolic disorder syndrome. The present article will review the progress in endocrine characteristics and regulatory mechanism of follicular development and ovulation failure in the mammalian ovary.

Keywords: follicle-stimulating hormone, follicular development, luteinizing hormone, ovulation failure, polycystic ovary syndrome

1. Introduction

In mammals, the follicular development mainly includes several periods of primordial follicles, primary follicles, secondary follicles, tertiary follicles, and matured follicles. With the initiation of primordial follicle, primary follicles are gradually formed, then continue to develop to the secondary and tertiary follicles, and finally to matured follicles, which were divided into two stages: the selective follicle stage and the matured follicle stage. The development of follicles undergoes the development of early stage, the growth of antral follicles, the selection of dominant follicles, the maturation, and ovulation of follicles. During an estrous cycle, when thousands of primordial follicles develop to the ovulation stage, the number of ovulation accounts for only 0.1–0.2% of the total number of primordial follicles. Most of these follicles are atresia during the development, while the hormone regulation is accompanied by the follicular development all the time. Pituitary gonadotropin and steroid hormones promote the growth of oocytes, the proliferation of the follicular cells, and the formation of the follicular cavity, which plays an important role in the follicular development. Polycystic ovary syndrome (PCOS) is an endocrine disorder syndrome with reproductive dysfunction and abnormal glucose metabolism in most PCOS women [1], and its clinical characteristics are large antral follicle pool from which to recruit and persistent anovulation. Further understanding the regulatory mechanism of the follicular development and ovulation in the ovaries will provide theoretical basis for the treatment of PCOS.

2. Hormonal regulation of the normal follicular development

Under physiological conditions, the growth and development of follicles are regulated by a variety of hormones, including pituitary gonadotropins (follicle-stimulating hormone, FSH and luteinizing hormone, LH) and gonadal hormones (estrogen and androgen). Androgen promotes the growth and development of early follicles [2] and plays an important role in the follicular recruitment [3]; FSH recruits the follicles [4] and LH binds to its receptors to promote the androgen synthesis in the follicular membrane cells; FSH binds to its receptors to activate the aromatase activity in the granulosa cells and then to promote the transformation of androgen to estradiol; estrogen promotes the growth and differentiation of follicular cells and cooperates with FSH to promote the development of the follicles; LH is secreted in a peak manner during the late follicular development for the ovulation of matured follicles.

2.1 Hormonal regulation of the early follicular development

It is generally believed that preantral follicles do not need the action of FSH, but studies have found that there are FSH receptors in the granulosa cells of preantral follicles, indicating that these follicles have the ability to respond to FSH very early. The threshold theory proposed by Brown in 1978 shows that the concentration of FSH is very important in the early follicle stage [5]. Once the FSH reaches the threshold, the follicle will enter the growth stage rapidly. The duration of FSH reaching the threshold and the extent of FSH exceeding the threshold will ultimately determine the number of matured follicles [5]. During the pre-antral follicular phase, inhibin-containing follicular fluid was injected into mice and cattle, which reduced the concentration of FSH, caused follicular growth to stop, and delayed the appearance of new follicular waves; and artificial increase of FSH concentration would lead to larger follicular volume and more follicles [6]. Therefore, FSH plays an important role in the initiation and development of primordial follicles during the follicular development [7].

LH receptor (LHR) is widely distributed in nongonadal tissues besides follicular endometrial cells and Leydig cells. The expression of LHR was later than that of FSH receptor (FSHR) [6, 8]. The expression of LHR mRNA could only be detected 5 days after the birth of the mouse offspring and 7 days after the birth of the rabbits when secondary follicles appeared in the ovaries [8]. In the estrous bovine and rabbit ovaries, LHR began to transcript in the follicular endometrial cells only after the follicles developed into antral follicles and follicular endometrium formed, and later in granulosa cells, indicating that LH had no direct effect on the development of preantral follicles.

2.2 Hormonal regulation of the antral follicles

After FSH initiates the development of primordial follicles, it further promotes the formation of some follicles into the cavity and enters the growth of antral follicles. The continuous growth of antral follicles depends on the support of FSH, while FSH stimulates the growth and development of antral follicles, and at the same time stimulates granulosa cells to produce FSHR. With the increase of the number of FSHR, the response of follicular granulosa cells to FSHR increases, which promotes the continuous development of granulosa cells [9].

Follicular intima began to synthesize LHR, cholesterol side chain cleavage enzyme (P450scc), P450 17alpha hydroxylase (P450 17alpha), and 3beta hydroxysteroid dehydrogenase (3beta-HSD) after the formation of antral follicles. The development of antral follicles is related to the synthesis of P450scc and P450arom enzymes by granulosa cells. LH acts on follicular endometrial cells, P450scc and 3beta-HSD catalyze the conversion of cholesterol to progesterone, and progesterone to androgen under the action of P450 17alpha and P450 C17,20 carbon chain lyase [10].

2.3 Hormonal regulation of the dominant follicles

Some of the first growing follicles were selected to continue to develop into dominant follicles. The remaining follicles in the same group were transformed into secondary follicles and gradually degenerated into atresia [11]. With the advent of dominant follicles, the concentration of FSH gradually decreased to the basic concentration and is maintained until the next peak. During the later selection period, the response ability of dominant follicles to FSH decreased, and the decrease of the peak value of FSH was obviously a necessary factor for the selection of dominant follicles, but not the only factor. LH also played an important role in this process.

During the selection process of dominant follicles, the number of FSH receptors in granulosa cells remained unchanged, while the expression of LHR mRNA was initial, and the number of LHR increased gradually [12]. At the same time, the number of LH binding sites in endometrial cells increased when the dominant follicle was established, so the selection of dominant follicles began to change from FSH dependent to LH dependent one, and the number of LH receptors increased rapidly.

Androgen enters granulosa cells, FSH acts on granulosa cells, induces the proliferation and differentiation of granulosa cells, and increases the activity of P450arom, which converts androgen into estrogen [11]. With the increase of estradiol produced by follicles, estradiol has a feedback effect on pituitary gonadotropin, which makes the concentration of gonadotropin decrease slightly, inhibits the development of other follicles, and promotes atresia of other follicles. In addition, FSH has long sensitization to aromatase [13].

Inhibin (INH) is a glycoprotein hormone produced mainly by ovarian granulosa cells. It is a heterodimer composed of two subunits, alpha and beta [14]. INH stimulates androstenedione synthesis in the follicular membrane mediated by LH and enhances aromatase activity, thus increasing estradiol synthesis in granulosa cells. It is of great significance for follicular recruitment and selection of superior follicles. After the formation of dominant follicles, INH and 17beta-estradiol synthesized by granulosa cells increased, and inhibited FSH synthesis and release by blood circulation. On the one hand, the decrease of FSH synthesis restricts the further development of non-dominant follicles and makes them become atresia follicles; on the other hand, INH enhances the sensitivity of dominant follicles to pituitary gonadotropin and avoids follicular stagnation caused by the decrease of FSH synthesis [15].

2.4 Hormonal regulation of ovulation

Ovulation in animals is a complex process, involving a series of changes such as the rupture of matured follicles and excretion of matured oocyte. The hormone that fundamentally affects ovulation is LH. After selecting the dominant follicles, the gonadotropin-dependent transformation was completed, and the estrogen in the follicles increased rapidly, with the peak value of estradiol [16]. With the emergence of estradiol peak, the pituitary response to gonadotropin-releasing hormone (GnRH) gradually increased, and the LH stored in pituitary increased in order to further provide hormones to the LH release pool, which reached the peak before ovulation. LH peak causes follicular wall ischemia to form a necrosis state of "physiological atrophy," leading to ovulation [9].

As in the case of LH, the concentration of FSH in blood increased briefly before ovulation and reached a peak again before ovulation. It is worth noting that LH must cooperate with a certain proportion of FSH in order to promote normal ovulation. LH ruptures all the follicles on the ovary, but when they are used together, only matured follicles are discharged, indicating that FSH has a mechanism to inhibit the rupture of immatured follicles.

The appearance of LH peak activates adenylate cyclase in the follicular membrane, increases cAMP, causes the luteinization of granulosa cells, increases progesterone content in the follicles, thus inhibits the positive feedback of estrogen to promote LH secretion [9], reduces the frequency of LH pulse [9], prolongs the duration of LH rise before ovulation, and ensures the sufficient time for LH and other gonadotropins to initiate follicular maturation and ovulation. At the same time, progesterone activates proteolytic enzymes, amylase, collagenase, and hyaluronidase in the follicles. These enzymes act on the collagen structure of the follicular wall to decrease the tension, increase the expansibility, and finally cause the ovulation.

INH acts as a chemical signal of the pituitary gland to induce the number of developing follicles in the ovary and reduce the release of FSH to maintain the level of species-specific ovulation [17]. Estradiol transmits chemical signals to the hypothalamus during the follicular maturation, so INH is an important inducer of the follicular development, which controls the number of follicles by inhibiting the release of FSH [18].

3. Endocrine regulation of the follicular development in PCOS

PCOS patients are predominantly androgens and the excessive androgens are mainly androstenedione and testosterone [19]. Recent studies have found that other endocrine factors are also involved in the occurrence of PCOS, such as leptin, growth hormone, and so on.

3.1 Androgen

The increase of androgen level in follicular fluid blocks the development of dominant follicles [20], while the main mechanism of androgen excess in PCOS is as following. LH directly acts on the follicular membrane cells, increases the activity of P450 C17 enzyme in the cells, and causes the excessive androgen production in the follicular membrane cells; high level of INS increases the level of LH in PCOS patients, thus promoting the secretion of androgen by ovaries and adrenal glands; insulin-like growth factor (IGF)-I promote androgen production in the follicular membrane cells and adrenal cortical cells; and adrenal hyperfunction also produces a large amount of dehydroepiandrosterone (DHEA) and dehydroepiandrosterone sulfate (DHEAS) [21].

3.2 Gonadotropin

The serum FSH level of PCOS patients was lower than that of normal people, but low FSH level resulted in a large number of follicles accumulated and could not develop into dominant follicles, resulting in anovulation and the changes of polycystic ovarian [22, 23]. Although the persistent high androgen level in the ovary of PCOS patients cannot form dominant follicles, the small follicles in the ovary can still secrete estradiol. At the same time, the increase of estrone converted from androstenedione in the peripheral blood makes the persistent secretion of large amounts of estrogen and a certain level of estradiol act on the hypothalamus and pituitary gland, which has a positive feedback effect on LH, and increases its secretion amplitude and frequency. The level of LH is continuously high, and then stimulates the hyperplasia of follicular membrane, produces excessive androgens, significantly inhibits the role of LH in promoting estradiol secretion, which may be the cause of oocyte maturation disorder in PCOS patients [24].

3.3 Insulin

Insulin (INS) receptors are expressed in ovarian stromal cells, granulosa cells, and follicular membrane cells. INS promotes the follicular recruitment and stimulates the synthesis of steroid hormones by follicular membrane cells and granulosa cells [25]. INS promotes androgen production by follicular membrane cells through the following pathways [26] and plays an important role in the production of hyperandrogenism [27]. INS increases androgen production by enhancing the activity of 17alpha-hydroxylase, increases androgen production by increasing the number of LH receptors or the affinity of LH to receptors, increases free androgen level by reducing the secretion of gonadal hormone binding globulin in the liver, and increases androgen level by inhibiting the secretion of IGF binding protein and enhancing the activity of serum IGF-I. INS resistance exists in PCOS patients, which leads to the hyperinsulinemia and increases androgen production and premature luteinization of granulosa cells, thus causing granulosa cell proliferation and follicular development to stagnate [26, 27].

3.4 Leptin

Leptin is a polypeptide hormone secreted by adipose tissue [28], which plays an important role in controlling reproductive capacity [29]. The disorder of leptin system is related to the pathogenesis of polycystic ovary [29–32]. Relatively high concentrations of leptin in serum and follicular fluid of PCOS patients resulted in lower fertilization, transfer, and pregnancy rates in vitro fertilization-embryo transfer (IVF-ET) [33]. The high concentration of leptin in PCOS patients inhibits the aromatase activity of granulosa cells, prevents the transformation of androgen to estrogen, induces hyperandrogenism, and inhibits follicular development [34]. In addition, leptin may block the selection and development of dominant follicles, leading to anovulation [35].

3.5 Growth hormone

Growth hormone (GH) is a hormone secreted by pituitary gland, which has physiological effects on the growth, development, and metabolism, which stimulates the follicular development, inhibits follicular atresia, and increases ovulation number [36]. GH directly regulates the gene expression of IGF-I or IGF-II and affects the synthesis of ovarian hormones. The impairment of GH secretion and the decrease of GH level lead to anovulation in PCOS. In addition, INS inhibits the secretion of pituitary GH stimulated by basal and gonadotropin-releasing hormone and also stimulates the production of IGF-II, thus feedback inhibits GH secretion [36].

4. Molecular mechanism regulating the follicular development

Follicular development is regulated by many molecules and related signaling pathways in mammals. For example, prematured luteinization of granulosa cells in mouse follicles is associated with higher LH levels in the follicles, which results in the early meiosis of oocyte and changes in signal transduction, leading to follicular atresia [37]. In addition, activin/inhibin, BMP/Smad, and NPPC/NPR2 signaling pathways also play an active role in the development of ovarian follicles, which will be discussed in the present section.

4.1 Activin/inhibin signaling pathway

Activin is an intercellular signaling molecule secreted mainly by granulosa cells, and also an agonist-stimulating pituitary gland secreting FSH. Activin is involved in many biological functions of mammalian ovaries, including the survival of germ cells and the recruitment of primordial follicles, promotes the proliferation of granulosa cells and the expression of FSHR, delays the luteinization and atresia of follicles, and participates in the luteolysis [38–40]. Activin binds to type II receptor, starts the phosphorylation process, then activates type I receptor, phosphorylates the downstream signal molecule R-Smads, receptor Smad binding to phosphorylated R-Smads occurs the location transfer, and enters into the nucleus to bind with specific receptors, playing a regulatory role. Activin also promotes the proliferation and activity of granulosa cells through smad2/ERK5 signaling pathway, increases the secretion of stem cell factor (SCF, also known as Kit ligand, KL), and then specifically binds to the surface receptor c-Kit of oocytes. The expression level of SCF/c-Kit in rat ovary after binding is increased, thus promoting the development of oocytes [38].

Inhibin is a kind of macromolecule glycoprotein hormone secreted by the gonad, and its structure is similar to activin. Inhibin regulates the synthesis and secretion of pituitary FSH together with activin [41, 42]. During the development stage of dominant follicles, the concentration of inhibin A increased, which increased the sensitivity of dominant follicles to FSH and prevented dominant follicles from atresia. During the luteal formation stage, inhibin A mainly promotes the luteinization of follicles, inhibin B mainly expresses in the small and medium follicles, and enhances FSH to prevent nondominant follicles from entering the preovulation stage, which was conducive to the screening of dominant follicles [43]. It was found that the level of inhibin B in the follicular fluid of PCOS patients decreased significantly [44].

4.2 BMP/Smad signaling pathway

The signal transduction of bone morphogenetic proteins (Bmps) family can be divided into two main pathways: Smads-dependent pathway and non-Smads-dependent pathway such as phosphatidylinositol 3 kinase (PI3K). Each member of the Smads family performs different functions in signal transduction pathways, which can be divided into three types: receptor-regulated Smads, CO-mediated Smads, and inhibitory Smads [45]. Bmps/Smads signaling pathway plays an important role in regulating follicular growth, granulosa cell growth and differentiation, oocyte maturation, and ovulation in mammals. Bmps bind to BMPR-II receptor on cell membrane and then make it phosphorylated. Phosphorylated BMPR-II receptor binds to BMP-I receptor to form a complex. BMP-I receptor is activated by corresponding protein kinase and phosphorylated. Then Smads signal molecule is activated. Activated R-Smads binding common CoSmad 4 forms Smad protein complex and enters the nucleus and specificity. DNA sequence binding start the promoter of downstream target gene, make downstream gene begin to transcribe [46–48], downstream signal molecule R-Smads also plays an important role in BMP/Smad signaling pathway. After Smad4 knockout, steroid hormone regulation was blocked, plasma progesterone level increased, and granulosa cells developed premature luteinization, which eventually led to premature ovarian failure [49].

4.3 NPPC/NPR2 signaling pathway

Natriuretic peptide family widely exists in animal brain, heart, and other tissues and organs, which has the functions of maintaining blood pressure and blood volume stability, promoting fat metabolism and cartilage growth. The family consists of three ligands and three specific receptors in mammals. Ligands exist in the form of precursor peptides, namely atrial natriuretic peptide (ANP, also known as NPPA), brain natriuretic peptide (BNP, also known as NPPB), C-type natriuretic peptide (CNP, also known as NPPC), and specific receptors exist in the form of dimers, namely natriuretic peptide receptor A (NPRA, also known as NPR1), natriuretic peptide receptor B (NPRB, also known as NPR2), and natriuretic peptide receptor C (NPRC, also known as NPR3) [50]. NPPC/NPR signaling pathway plays an important role in inhibiting premature maturation of mammalian oocytes. The combination of NPPC and NPR2 produced by granulosa cells of the follicular parietal layer stimulates the production of cGMP, which enters into the oocyte through interstitial links between oocyte and granulosa cells [51], inhibits the activity of phosphodiesterase (PDE3A), and decreases the degree of hydrolysis of cAMP, thus stabilizing at a higher level. The protein kinase PKA dependent on cAMP regulates the activity of maturation-promoting factor (MPF) through phosphatase cell division cycle 25 (CDC25), Wee1 kinase, and myelin transcription factor Myt1. CDC25 dephosphorylated cyclin-dependent kinase 1 (CDK1), Wee1 and Myt1 phosphorylated CDK1, phosphorylated CDK1 and related complexes inactivated, and ultimately inhibited the maturation of oocytes.

5. Conclusion

Nowadays, great achievements have been made in the molecular mechanism of follicular development in mammals. At present, many signaling pathways have been proved to play a very important role during the follicular growth and development, and some of them have been thoroughly studied. However, there are still some problems related to signaling pathways, such as how mammals initiate primordial follicular development and which downstream target genes are involved in signaling pathways. Follicular dysplasia in PCOS patients is closely related to apoptosis of granulosa cells, follicular atresia, and oocyte degeneration. Its mechanism is related to endocrine dysfunction, as well as regulation factors and their receptors in the ovary. Although PCOS patients can obtain a large number of oocytes, the low rate of matured oocytes, the low rate of high-quality embryos, the low pregnancy rate, and the high abortion rate make clear the related factors of oocyte degeneration and atresia regulation, which is of great significance to the application of assisted reproductive technology in PCOS patients. Therefore, further understanding the molecular mechanism regulating the follicular development in mammals still requires further study on the biology and gene expressions related to the follicular development, which is of great significance for the treatment of mammalian reproductive infertility and other diseases.

Acknowledgements

This study was supported by Fujian Provincial Natural Science Foundation (2017J01626 and 2018J01722), Fujian Province Science and Technology Project of The Education Department (JAT160118), and the Educational Reform Project (Y201809 and P201801016), the Science and Technology Innovation Project of Xi Yuan Jiang Program (FZSKG2018002), and the College Students' Innovation Training Project (CXXL2019268 and CXXL 2019274) of Fujian Normal University.

Conflict of interest

The authors declare no conflict of interests.

Author details

Zhenghong Zhang*, Yan Zhang, Fengping Lin and Zhengchao Wang
Provincial Key Laboratory for Developmental Biology and Neurosciences, College of Life Sciences, Fujian Normal University, Fuzhou, China

*Address all correspondence to: zhangzh@fjnu.edu.cn

References

[1] Wang F, Zhang ZH, Xiao KZ, Wang ZC. Roles of hypothalamic-pituitary-adrenal axis and hypothalamus-pituitary-ovary axis in the abnormal endocrine functions in patients with polycystic ovary syndrome. Zhongguo Yi Xue Ke Xue Yuan Xue Bao. 2017;**39**(5):699-704. DOI: 10.3881/j.issn.1000-503X.2017.05.017

[2] Abbott DH, Dumesic DA, Levine JE. Hyperandrogenic origins of polycystic ovary syndrome—Implications for pathophysiology and therapy. Expert Review of Endocrinology and Metabolism. 2019;**14**(2):131-143. DOI: 10.1080/17446651.2019.1576522

[3] Steckler T, Wang J, Bartol FF, Roy SK, Padmanabhan V. Fetal programming: Prenatal testosterone treatment causes intrauterine growth retardation, reduces ovarian reserve and increases ovarian follicular recruitment. Endocrinology. 2005;**146**(7):3185-3193. DOI: 10.1210/en.2004-1444

[4] Gougeon A. Regulation of ovarian follicular development in primates: Facts and hypotheses. Endocrine Reviews. 1996;**17**(2):121-155. DOI: 10.1210/edrv-17-2-121

[5] van Weissenbruch MM, Schoemaker HC, Drexhage HA, Schoemaker J. Pharmaco-dynamics of human menopausal gonadotrophin (HMG) and follicle-stimulating hormone (FSH). The importance of the FSH concentration in initiating follicular growth in polycystic ovary-like disease. Human Reproduction. 1993;**8**(6):813-821. DOI: 10.1093/oxfordjournals.humrep.a138147

[6] Fortune JE. Ovarian follicular growth and development in mammals. Biology of Reproduction. 1994;**50**(2):225-232. DOI: 10.1095/biolreprod50.2.225

[7] Campbell BK, Scaramuzzi RJ, Webb R. Control of antral follicle development and selection in sheep and cattle. Journal of Reproduction and Fertility. Supplement. 1995;**49**:335-350

[8] O'Shaughnessy PJ, McLelland D, McBride MW. Regulation of luteinizing hormone-receptor and follicle-stimulating hormone-receptor messenger ribonucleic acid levels during development in the neonatal mouse ovary. Biology of Reproduction. 1997;**57**(3):602-608. DOI: 10.1095/biolreprod57.3.602

[9] Wang Z, Shi F, Jiang YQ, Lu LZ, Wang H, Watanabe G, et al. Changes of cyclic AMP levels and phosphodiesterase activities in the rat ovary. The Journal of Reproduction and Development. 2007;**53**(4):717-725

[10] Bakhtyukov AA, Shpakov AO. The molecular mechanisms of steroidogenesis regulation in leydig cells. Tsitologiia. 2016;**58**(9):666-678

[11] Amsterdam A, Plehn-Dujowich D, Suh BS. Structure-function relationships during differentiation of normal and oncogene-transformed granulosa cells. Biology of Reproduction. 1992;**46**(4):513-522. DOI: 10.1095/biolreprod46.4.513

[12] Bodensteiner KJ, Wiltbank MC, Bergfelt DR, Ginther OJ. Alterations in follicular estradiol and gonadotropin receptors during development of bovine antral follicles. Theriogenology. 1996;**45**(2):499-512

[13] Hillier SG, Reichert LE Jr, Van Hall EV. Control of preovulatory follicular estrogen biosynthesis in the human ovary. The Journal of Clinical Endocrinology and Metabolism. 1981;**52**(5):847-856. DOI: 10.1210/jcem-52-5-847

[14] Burger HG. Inhibin: Definition and nomenclature, including related substances. The Journal of Endocrinology. 1988;**117**(2):159-160

[15] Evans AC, Komar CM, Wandji SA, Fortune JE. Changes in androgen secretion and luteinizing hormone pulse amplitude are associated with the recruitment and growth of ovarian follicles during the luteal phase of the bovine estrous cycle. Biology of Reproduction. 1997;**57**(2):394-401. DOI: 10.1095/biolreprod57.2.394

[16] Qvist R, Blackwell LF, Bourne H, Brown JB. Development of mouse ovarian follicles from primary to preovulatory stages in vitro. Journal of Reproduction and Fertility. 1990;**89**(1):169-180

[17] Nagata S, Miyake YI, Nambo Y, Nagamine N, Watanabe G, Tsunoda N, et al. Inhibin secretion in the stallion. Equine Veterinary Journal. 1998;**30**(2):98-103

[18] Kogo H, Takasaki K, Takeo S, Watanabe G, Taya K, Sasamoto S. Inhibition by indomethacin of the already accelerated secretion of inhibin and estradiol in equine chorionic gonadotropin-primed immature female rats. Biological & Pharmaceutical Bulletin. 1993;**16**(5):483-485

[19] Lainas TG, Petsas GK, Zorzovilis IZ, Iliadis GS, Lainas GT, Cazlaris HE, et al. Initiation of GnRH antagonist on Day 1 of stimulation as compared to the long agonist protocol in PCOS patients. A randomized controlled trial: Effect on hormonal levels and follicular development. Human Reproduction. 2007;**22**(6):1540-1546. DOI: 10.1093/humrep/dem033

[20] Kurzawa R, Ciepiela P, Baczkowski T, Safranow K, Brelik P. Comparison of embryological and clinical outcome in GnRH antagonist vs. GnRH agonist protocols for in vitro fertilization in PCOS non-obese patients. A prospective randomized study. Journal of Assisted Reproduction and Genetics. 2008;**25**(8):365-374. DOI: 10.1007/s10815-008-9249-7

[21] Silfen ME, Manibo AM, Ferin M, McMahon DJ, Levine LS, Oberfield SE. Elevated free IGF-I levels in prepubertal Hispanic girls with premature adrenarche: Relationship with hyperandrogenism and insulin sensitivity. The Journal of Clinical Endocrinology and Metabolism. 2002;**87**(1):398-403. DOI: 10.1210/jcem.87.1.8143

[22] Franks S, Stark J, Hardy K. Follicle dynamics and anovulation in polycystic ovary syndrome. Human Reproduction Update. 2008;**14**(4):367-378. DOI: 10.1093/humupd/dmn015

[23] Hillier SG. Current concepts of the roles of follicle stimulating hormone and luteinizing hormone in folliculogenesis. Human Reproduction. 1994;**9**(2):188-191. DOI: 10.1093/oxfordjournals.humrep.a138480

[24] Greisen S, Ledet T, Ovesen P. Effects of androstenedione, insulin and luteinizing hormone on steroidogenesis in human granulosa luteal cells. Human Reproduction. 2001;**16**(10):2061-2065. DOI: 10.1093/humrep/16.10.2061

[25] Kezele PR, Nilsson EE, Skinner MK. Insulin but not insulin-like growth factor-1 promotes the primordial to primary follicle transition. Molecular and Cellular Endocrinology. 2002;**192**(1-2):37-43

[26] Dumesic DA, Abbott DH. Implications of polycystic ovary syndrome on oocyte development. Seminars in Reproductive Medicine. 2008;**26**(1):53-61. DOI: 10.1055/s-2007-992925

[27] Pasquali R, Gambineri A. Insulin-sensitizing agents in women with

polycystic ovary syndrome. Fertility and Sterility. 2006;**86**(Suppl 1):S28-S29. DOI: 10.1016/j.fertnstert.2006.04.012

[28] Zhang Y, Proenca R, Maffei M, Barone M, Leopold L, Friedman JM. Positional cloning of the mouse obese gene and its human homologue. Nature. 1994;**372**(6505):425-432. DOI: 10.1038/372425a0

[29] Goumenou AG, Matalliotakis IM, Koumantakis GE, Panidis DK. The role of leptin in fertility. European Journal of Obstetrics, Gynecology, and Reproductive Biology. 2003;**106**(2):118-124

[30] Pasquali R, Gambineri A, Cavazza C, Ibarra Gasparini D, Ciampaglia W, Cognigni GE, et al. Heterogeneity in the responsiveness to long-term lifestyle intervention and predictability in obese women with polycystic ovary syndrome. European Journal of Endocrinology. 2011;**164**(1):53-60. DOI: 10.1530/EJE-10-0692

[31] Polak K, Czyzyk A, Simoncini T, Meczekalski B. New markers of insulin resistance in polycystic ovary syndrome. Journal of Endocrinological Investigation. 2017;**40**(1):1-8. DOI: 10.1007/s40618-016-0523-8

[32] Chen CI, Hsu MI, Lin SH, Chang YC, Hsu CS, Tzeng CR. Adiponectin and leptin in overweight/obese and lean women with polycystic ovary syndrome. Gynecological Endocrinology. 2015;**31**(4):264-268. DOI: 10.3109/09513590.2014.984676

[33] Li MG, Ding GL, Chen XJ, Lu XP, Dong LJ, Dong MY, et al. Association of serum and follicular fluid leptin concentrations with granulosa cell phosphorylated signal transducer and activator of transcription 3 expression in fertile patients with polycystic ovarian syndrome. The Journal of Clinical Endocrinology and Metabolism. 2007;**92**(12):4771-4776. DOI: 10.1210/jc.2007-0978

[34] Janeckova R. The role of leptin in human physiology and pathophysiology. Physiological Research. 2001;**50**(5):443-459

[35] Agarwal SK, Vogel K, Weitsman SR, Magoffin DA. Leptin antagonizes the insulin-like growth factor-I augmentation of steroidogenesis in granulosa and theca cells of the human ovary. The Journal of Clinical Endocrinology and Metabolism. 1999;**84**(3):1072-1076. DOI: 10.1210/jcem.84.3.5543

[36] Li XL, Wang L, Lv F, Huang XM, Wang LP, Pan Y, et al. The influence of different growth hormone addition protocols to poor ovarian responders on clinical outcomes in controlled ovary stimulation cycles: A systematic review and meta-analysis. Medicine (Baltimore). 2017;**96**(12):e6443. DOI: 10.1097/MD.0000000000006443

[37] Schwartz JC, Younger ST, Nguyen NB, Hardy DB, Monia BP, Corey DR, et al. Antisense transcripts are targets for activating small RNAs. Nature Structural & Molecular Biology. 2008;**15**(8):842-848

[38] Knight PG, Satchell L, Glister C. Intra-ovarian roles of activins and inhibins. Molecular and Cellular Endocrinology. 2012;**359**(1-2):53-65. DOI: 10.1016/j.mce.2011.04.024

[39] Xia Y, Schneyer AL. The biology of activin: Recent advances in structure, regulation and function. The Journal of Endocrinology. 2009;**202**(1):1-12. DOI: 10.1677/JOE-08-0549

[40] McLaughlin M, Bromfield JJ, Albertini DF, Telfer EE. Activin promotes follicular integrity and oogenesis in cultured pre-antral bovine follicles. Molecular Human Reproduction. 2010;**16**(9):644-653. DOI: 10.1093/molehr/gaq021

[41] Dan X, Liu X, Han Y, Liu Q, Yang L. Effect of the novel DNA vaccine

fusing inhibin α(1-32) and the RF-amide related peptide-3 genes on immune response, hormone levels and fertility in tan sheep. Animal Reproduction Science. 2016;**164**:105-110. DOI: 10.1016/j.anireprosci.2015.11.018

[42] Liu Q, Rehman ZU, Liu JJ, Han L, Liu XR, Yang LG. Nasal immunization with inhibin DNA vaccine delivered by attenuated salmonella choleraesuis for improving ovarian responses and fertility in cross-bred buffaloes. Reproduction in Domestic Animals. 2017;**52**(2):189-194. DOI: 10.1111/rda.12876

[43] Welt CK. Regulation and function of inhibins in the normal menstrual cycle. Seminars in Reproductive Medicine. 2004;**22**(3):187-193. DOI: 10.1055/s-2004-831894

[44] Welt CK, Taylor AE, Fox J, Messerlian GM, Adams JM, Schneyer AL. Follicular arrest in polycystic ovary syndrome is associated with deficient inhibin A and B biosynthesis. The Journal of Clinical Endocrinology and Metabolism. 2005;**90**(10):5582-5587. DOI: 10.1210/jc.2005-0695

[45] Pouliot F, Labrie C. Expression profile of agonistic smads in human breast cancer cells: Absence of regulation by estrogens. International Journal of Cancer. 1999;**81**(1):98-103

[46] Drummond AE. TGFbeta signalling in the development of ovarian function. Cell and Tissue Research. 2005;**322**(1):107-115. DOI: 10.1007/s00441-005-1153-1

[47] Yokota Y, Mori S. Role of Id family proteins in growth control. Journal of Cellular Physiology. 2002;**190**(1):21-28. DOI: 10.1002/jcp.10042

[48] Henningfeld KA, Friedle H, Rastegar S, Knöchel W. Autoregulation of Xvent-2B; direct interaction and functional cooperation of Xvent-2 and Smad1. The Journal of Biological Chemistry. 2002;**277**(3):2097-2103. DOI: 10.1074/jbc.M108524200

[49] Pangas SA, Li X, Robertson EJ, Matzuk MM. Premature luteinization and cumulus cell defects in ovarian-specific Smad4 knockout mice. Molecular Endocrinology. 2006;**20**(6):1406-1422. DOI: 10.1210/me.2005-0462

[50] Dickey DM, Yoder AR, Potter LR. A familial mutation renders atrial natriuretic peptide resistant to proteolytic degradation. The Journal of Biological Chemistry. 2009;**284**(29):19196-19202. DOI: 10.1074/jbc.M109.010777

[51] Norris RP, Ratzan WJ, Freudzon M, Mehlmann LM, Krall J, Movsesian MA, et al. Cyclic GMP from the surrounding somatic cells regulates cyclic AMP and meiosis in the mouse oocyte. Development. 2009;**136**(11):1869-1878. DOI: 10.1242/dev.035238

Chapter 6

Expression and Contribution of Insulin Signaling Pathway to the Development of Polycystic Ovary Syndrome

Qingqiang Lin, Hong Zhang, Jiuhua Zhao and Zhengchao Wang

Abstract

Our previous studies have demonstrated that insulin signaling pathway has an important role in the pathophysiology of polycystic ovary syndrome (PCOS), including phosphatidylinositol 3-kinase and protein kinase B signaling, which is critically implicated in insulin resistance, androgen secretion, obesity, and follicular development. PCOS manifests as defective ovarian steroid biosynthesis and hyperandrogenemia, and 50–70% of women with PCOS exhibit insulin resistance and are hyperinsulinemic, indicating that insulin resistance and hyperinsulinism may have an important role in the pathophysiology of PCOS. Therefore, the present article will review the contribution of insulin signaling pathway to the abnormal regulation of follicular growth and ovulation, which can cause corresponding reproductive endocrine diseases and affect women's reproductive health. Exploring the mechanism of insulin signaling pathway in PCOS will help not only to understand the physiology and pathology of follicular development but also to provide theoretical basis for the treatment of PCOS.

Keywords: insulin receptor substrates, protein kinase B, hypoxia-inducible factor-1, granulosa cells, polycystic ovary syndrome

1. Introduction

Polycystic ovary syndrome (PCOS) is an endocrine disorder syndrome with reproductive dysfunction and abnormal glucose metabolism, which is characterized by excessive androgen. It is usually accompanied by insulin resistance (IR) and is also a most common endocrine disorder in women of reproductive age [1]. Although the exact cause of PCOS is not clear, it belongs to endocrine and metabolic diseases. It has been concluded that there are not only endocrine disorders but also metabolic abnormalities with many subtypes. Burghen firstly proposed that insulin resistance (IR) was involved in the pathogenesis of PCOS in 1980 [2], and a large number of studies have subsequently confirmed the close relationship between IR and PCOS. IR is a metabolic state in which the normal insulin-promoted glucose uptake and utilization decreased and the compensatory insulin secretion from tissues and organs of the body maintained the stability of blood glucose.

Clinically, PCOS presents after puberty menarche, and patients have the abnormal glucose metabolism and the pathophysiology related to the physiological changes of puberty. IR is not only a normal physiological change of adolescent girls but also an important pathophysiological change of PCOS, that is, IR and compensatory hyperinsulinemia. IR is one of the important pathophysiological mechanisms in the occurrence and development of many PCOS and also an important cause of hyperandrogenism and ovarian dysfunction.

2. Historical overview

The defect of insulin signaling pathway is one of the important mechanisms of PCOS after two centuries of research, and the historical development process is summarized as the following [2–11]. Achard and Thiers firstly described the relationship between abnormal glucose metabolism and hyperandrogenism in 1921, and Kierland et al. believed that hyperandrogenism was related to higher incidence of acanthosis nigricans in female patients with diabetes mellitus in 1947. Kahn et al. mainly focused on the relationship between the abnormal metabolism in the adolescent and the hyperandrogenism, insulin resistance, and acanthosis nigricans in the postmenopausal women in 1976 and believed the postmenopausal pathogens are caused by the result of endogenous IR and the onset of adolescent women is caused by the mutation of insulin receptor. Until 1980, Burghen et al. reported that hyperinsulinemia is closely related to PCOS for the first time and found that hyperinsulinemia existed in PCOS patients with hyperandrogenism under the basal state and after glucose stimulation compared with normal people of the same age and weight, suggesting IR existed and insulin was highly correlated with androgen levels. During the mid-1980s, Dunaif et al. found the follicular membrane cells of typical PCOS women proliferated significantly and the morphological changes of their hyperplasia were more common in PCOS patients with IR, suggesting that hyperinsulinemia affected ovarian morphology and functions.

3. Pathological changes and clinical characteristics of PCOS

Typical polycystic ovaries have stromal hypertrophy, and their volume is 2 times larger than that of normal ovaries. The ovaries showed bilateral sclerosing polycystic degeneration and gray-white or oyster-colored [12]. There is "strand of pearls" appearance on USN, 2-7 mm diameter cystic follicles or large retention follicular cysts under the capsule. Microscopic examination showed atresia follicles increased, no matured follicles formed, cortical surface fibrosis, fewer cells, obvious blood vessels, a large number of outer follicles luteinized, and no signs of ovulation.

Menstrual disorders are the main manifestations of adolescent PCOS patients, with common symptoms such as hirsutism, acne, and body mass increase [12]. But these symptoms can also be the normal physiological manifestations after puberty, so most patients continue to see a doctor for infertility after several years. In addition to the physical changes caused by infertility and excessive androgens, the metabolic syndrome is more prone to cause, mainly including androgenism and metabolic abnormalities such as insulin, glucose, and lipid. Hypertension is more common in the late stage, and cardiovascular diseases such as type 2 diabetes mellitus and coronary heart disease are induced. Many PCOS patients often have IR and hyperinsulinemia as the first manifestation, followed by excessive androgen and reproductive dysfunction.

4. Insulin signaling pathway

Insulin is a multifunctional protein polypeptide, which binds to its specific insulin receptor and causes a series of signal amplification cascade reactions with two main signaling pathways; one is the phosphatidylinositol 3 kinase/protein kinase B (PI3K/PKB) pathway, and the other is the mitogen-activated protein kinase/extracellular signal-regulated kinase (MAPK/ERK) pathway. These two signaling pathways are related to the self-phosphorylation of tyrosine residues in receptors, and insulin mainly mediates its metabolic regulation through PI3K pathway [3, 13–16].

PI3K is a kind of kinase that catalyzes phosphatidylinositol, which can be activated by receptor tyrosine kinase or G protein-coupled receptor. It consists of a catalytic subunit P110 and an inhibitory regulatory subunit p85, and it has the activity of lipid kinase and serine/threonine protein kinase. Many growth factors, such as insulin, insulin-like growth factor (IGF), platelet-derived growth factor (PDGF), and epidermal growth factor (EGF), bind to the corresponding receptors; then tyrosine phosphorylation of the receptor itself and binding of p85 to the phosphorylated receptors relieve the inhibitory effect on p110, and PI3K is then activated. PKB is a member of the serine/threonine protein kinase family and a direct target protein downstream of PI3K. The phosphorylation of 308-site threonine (Thr308) and 473-site serine (Ser473) required for complete activation of AKT depends on PI3K catalysis. After the activation of PI3K/PKB pathway, PI3K/PKB pathway acts on a variety of substrates, mainly regulating the material metabolism of cells, besides participating in cell survival and anti-apoptosis. After insulin binds to insulin receptor alpha subunit located in the cellular membrane, it further triggers tyrosine phosphorylation of beta subunit itself and further phosphorylates tyrosine subunit of insulin receptor substrate (IRS). p-IRS can further activate PI3K and then produce PIP3, a second messenger. PIP3 binds to signal proteins PKB and phosphoinositide dependent kinase-1 (PDK1), which contain the PH domain in cells, and assists PDK1 to phosphorylate 308-site threonine of PKB to make it an active form. Activated-PKB can promote the transfer of glucose carrier-4 (GLUT-4) from the cytoplasm to the envelope and promote the absorption of glucose. PKB then phosphorylates tuberous sclerosis complex protein 1/2 (TSC1/2) to the inactive state, releases its inhibition on the downstream Rheb-GDP, converts it into Rheb-GTP, and further activates target of rapamycin complex 1 (TORC1). In addition, PKB also phosphorylates PRAS40, an inhibitor of mTORC1, to separate it from mTORC1, thereby activating mTORC1 and further exerting downstream cascade reactions, such as hypoxia-inducible factor-alpha (HIF-1alpha)/endothelin-2 (ET-2) signaling pathway-dependent ovulation [3, 13–16].

5. Insulin resistance and polycystic ovary syndrome

Insulin resistance is the defect of insulin signaling transduction, and PI3K/PKB signaling pathway is the main signaling pathway of insulin. In the state of IR, the role of PI3K signaling pathway induced by insulin stimulation decreased [3, 13]. The factors leading to abnormal insulin signaling transduction can be divided into congenital factors and acquired factors. Inborn abnormal factors, such as genetic defect and gene mutation, and other acquired factors, like lifestyle, obesity, and environment, can all cause IR by affecting PI3K/PKB signaling pathway. It was found that with the increase of free fatty acids in blood, they were converted into acy-CoA, DAG was increased, PKC was activated, serine residues in IRS-1 were phosphorylated, tyrosine phosphorylation in IRS-1 was decreased, PI3K activation was disturbed, and GLUT4 translocation to cell surface was affected, thus reducing insulin-mediated glucose utilization [3, 13, 17]. The increase of free fatty acids leads to the increase of lipids in muscle, which in turn interferes with the use and storage of insulin to glucose and causes IR.

PCOS patients had no significant difference in insulin receptor quantity and binding ability compared with non-PCOS patients, but the phosphorylation of insulin receptor decreased in PCOS patients, and the maximum glucose transport rate stimulated by insulin decreased [11, 18]. PCOS patients often have IR and hyperandrogenism, and IR plays a greater role in the formation of hyperandrogenism, while hyperandrogenism has no significant effect on the formation of IR. IR is the biological effect of insulin produced at physiological level in the body, which is lower than the actual level. The effect of insulin in promoting the absorption and utilization of glucose by organs, tissues, and cells is reduced, that is, the insulin sensitivity of tissues is reduced [3, 19, 20]. Hyperinsulinemia is a marker that insulin regulates glycometabolism in the compensatory stage under the state of IR [3, 19, 20].

At the cellular level, IR means that insulin signaling transduction is blocked or weakened. This signaling from insulin receptor down to the end-mediated substrates of insulin action involves many aspects of cell metabolism [3, 17–20]. Any link of insulin signaling impairment can lead to IR, which is closely related to the impairment of key molecules in the signaling of insulin, insulin receptor, insulin receptor substrate, PI3K, and GLUT4, specifically divided into the following three aspects [3, 17–20]: First, pre-receptor IR. The mutation of insulin gene leads to the changes of insulin primary structure and the decrease of biological activity, resulting in body IR. Secondly, receptor-level IR. The mutation of insulin receptor gene, which cannot be cleaved into matured alpha and beta receptor subunits, reduced the biosynthesis of insulin receptor or the affinity between insulin receptor and insulin, resulting in the loss of intracellular effect of insulin and leading to IR. Lastly, post-receptor IR. Insulin deficiency refers to a series of abnormal metabolic processes that occur when insulin binds to receptors and transmits signals to cells, which is the main cause of IR in PCOS patients. The physiological effect of insulin on glucose is the result of key enzyme activation such as insulin-dependent GLUT4 and G-kinase and glycogen synthase, and the defects in the structure or function of these enzymes can lead to IR [3, 13, 17–21]. Increased serine phosphorylation of insulin receptor may weaken the tyrosine kinase activity of insulin receptor, which may be the mechanism of post-receptor deficiency in PCOS patients.

6. PCOS ovarian IR

It is still controversial whether PCOS is a reflection of ovarian hypersensitivity to insulin or whether systemic IR is localized in ovaries. The study found that PCOS patients secrete more androgens than normal women after insulin stimulation. In addition, PCOS patients with normal insulin levels were treated with insulin sensitizers, and it was found that insulin levels decreased slowly and ovarian androgen levels also decreased [22].

6.1 Molecular mechanism of IR in the follicular membrane cells of PCOS

The most common symptoms of PCOS patients are excessive androgens in the ovary, especially increased testosterone production by follicular membrane cells. Insulin can stimulate the activity of steroid hormones in follicular theca cells through a variety of ways, one of which is through the MAPK pathway, which is still controversial; the other is through LH to induce the accumulation of cyclic adenosine phosphate (cAMP), which stimulates the activity of PI3K [23]. Studies have shown that LH and insulin have synergistic effects on the gene expression and mRNA accumulation of steroid hormone acute synthesis rapid regulatory protein (StAR) and cytochrome P450c17 (CYP-17). The increased PKB phosphorylation in insulin signaling pathway promotes the production of PCOS clinical symptoms such as follicular cell proliferation, follicular dysplasia, or anovulation, suggesting that insulin induces the synthesis of steroid hormones in follicular cells, which may be regulated by PI3K pathway, and PKB is a downstream regulator of this pathway [24–26]. A special blocker (LY294002) was used to block the PI3K pathway, which inhibited the activation of PKB and weakened the activity of 17a-hydroxylase and also proved the above opinion [26].

6.2 Molecular mechanism of IR in the granulosa cells of PCOS

Insulin can increase the activity of LDL receptor transcription factors through intracellular mechanisms such as protein kinase A (PKA), PI3K, and MAPK signaling pathways, thus promoting steroid hormone synthesis [27]. It has been found that after inhibiting PI3K with wortmannin, IR is produced by interfering with the intracellular glycometabolic signaling pathway [26]. Franks compared anovulatory PCOS patients with ovulatory PCOS patients and found the abnormal glucose metabolism in granulosa cells and the significantly impaired insulin-stimulated lactate production, while insulin-mediated glucose metabolism was resisted besides the steroid hormone secretion remaining normal. Therefore, the complex mechanism of insulin deficiency can also be found in the local of the ovary [28]. Our previous studies further found that PI3K/PKB signaling pathway was impaired in PCOS granulosa cells, which affected the downstream HIF-1a/ET-2-dependent ovulation mechanism, leading to PCOS anovulation [13, 29, 30].

7. Effects of IR on ovarian functions

Insulin can activate or inhibit ovarian hormone synthase and stimulate steroid hormone synthesis in ovarian cells with the species or cell specificity. Human ovarian matrix and follicles have insulin receptor distribution and can produce IGF and binding protein. Therefore, the ovary is one of the important target organs of insulin [7–9].

7.1 Effect of IR on the level of androgen hormone

Insulin enhances the binding ability of LH by increasing the LH receptor of granulosa cells; insulin acts on the pituitary gland to increase the sensitivity of gonadotropin-releasing hormone (GnRH); insulin inhibits the synthesis of sex hormone-binding protein in the liver and increases the level of free insulin [7–9]. PCOS patients taking insulin sensitizer can increase the binding protein in the circulation and decrease the free hormone, thus alleviating hyperandrogenism caused by hyperinsulinemia or IR [7–9].

7.2 Effect of IR on the proliferation of granulosa cells

The proliferation and physiological function of ovarian granulosa cells are very important for the follicular maturation and ovulation, while FSH, IGF2, and insulin are important factors to promote the proliferation of granulosa cells. In PCOS patients, insulin regulates the glucose uptake of ovarian granulosa cells, and the synthesis of lactic acid, a metabolite of glucose utilization, significantly decreases, resulting in the impaired insulin metabolism [7–9]. Insulin can induce IR and affect the proliferation of granulosa cells in PCOS patients, and most of the PCOS patients are complicated with hyperinsulinemia, high insulin concentration in the follicular fluid. However, the proliferation of granulosa cells was inhibited, and apoptosis was increased. Both of them synergistically enhance the expression of LH and HCG receptors in granulosa cells. The granulosa cells with 50–100 μm follicles have acquired the function of LH receptors only in matured follicles with a diameter of about 20 μm during normal menstrual cycle, which makes the granulosa cells with lumen follicle stage prematurely luteinized and inhibits their proliferation, leading to follicular stagnation [7–9]. Insulin also strengthens the response of granulosa cells to LH, leading to the LH-like peak at the elevated level of LH, which leads to the arrest of granulosa cell proliferation, follicular growth arrest, and anovulation [28].

7.3 Effect of IR on the development of ovarian follicles

Intraovarian follicular development undergoes a series of physiological processes, such as recruitment, selection, dominance, and ovulation. The basic manifestations of follicular dysplasia in PCOS patients are excessive follicular recruitment, blocked follicular selection and dominance, follicular stagnation, and anovulation [7–9]. Hyperinsulinemia in PCOS patients increases the sensitivity of preantral follicles to FSH, leading to excessive follicular recruitment, androgen synthesis in thecal cells, and conversion to estradiol. Furthermore, estradiol decreased the secretion of pituitary FSH due to negative feedback regulation, and the follicles lacked FSH stimulation and grew slowly, leading to the accumulation of preantral follicles and small sinusoidal follicles. The immaturity of follicles resulted in the accumulation of a large number of sinusoidal follicles and the formation of a unique polycystic ovary [31, 32]. Insulin is also one of the most powerful factors affecting plasma plasminogen activator inhibitor-1 (PAI-1). Hyperinsulinemia causes the excessive PAI-1 production in the liver and inhibits the ovulation by inhibiting the conversion of plasminogen to plasmin. The effects of hyperinsulinemia and IGF-2 on ovarian primordial follicles were continuously activated and finally formed the characteristic ovarian morphological changes of PCOS [33, 34].

7.4 Effect of IR on the signaling of ovarian PI3K

In the IR state, the decrease of PI3K signaling induced by insulin leads to the abnormal insulin signaling transduction. PI3K signaling is mainly related to the regulation of insulin on glucose metabolism. The signal molecule downstream of IRS is the key protein for insulin signaling to regulate the glucose metabolism. Activated PI3K, on the one hand, triggers vesicles rich in GLUT4 to translocate to the cell surface through the form of exocytosis from the endokaryon via Golgi apparatus, increases GLUT4 on the cell surface, and regulates the uptake of glucose by myocytes, adipocytes, and hepatocytes. On the other hand, activated PI3K inhibits gluconeogenesis by inhibiting enol pyruvate carboxykinase and ultimately increases the utilization of glucose and glycogen [7–9, 28]. Our previous studies have clearly demonstrated that the mechanism of IR in PCOS ovaries is related to post-insulin receptor signaling disorder [13, 29, 30]. At the same time, IR is also a key link in the pathogenesis of PCOS, so the causal relationship between PCOS and IR is still unclear.

8. Conclusion

PCOS is a disease involving many factors such as heredity and environment, and IR plays an important role in the development of PCOS. After insulin binds to receptors, it exerts its biological effects through a series of signaling pathways. Obstacles in any link of the pathways can lead to the signaling disorders and cause IR. Compensatory hyperinsulinemia and IR are considered to be the pathological basis of abnormal glucose metabolism and reproductive dysfunction in PCOS patients. Although the signaling pathway of insulin and its mechanism during the occurrence and development of insulin resistance are still poorly understood, PI3K/PKB pathway, as the main signal pathway of insulin, is involved in the metabolism of glucose and lipid in vivo. Further study about the regulatory mechanism of PI3K/PKB pathway and the interaction between the molecule and targeted molecule is needed and has high clinical value and application prospects to develop PI3K/Akt signaling pathway-specific drugs as a new target of IR therapy. At the same time, using modern molecular biology technology to comprehensively understand insulin signaling pathway and in-depth study of IR molecular mechanism of PCOS can provide a solid theoretical basis for clinical diagnosis and treatment.

Acknowledgements

This study was supported by National Training Program of Innovation and Entrepreneurship for Undergraduates (201910394023), Fujian Provincial Natural Science Foundation (2017J01626 and 2018J01722), Fujian Province Science and Technology Project of The Education Department (JAT160118), and the Educational Reform Project (Y201809 and P201801016), the Science and Technology Innovation Project of Xi Yuan Jiang Program (FZSKG2018002), and Training Program of Innovation and Entrepreneurship for Undergraduates (CXXL2019268 and CXXL 2019274) of Fujian Normal University. Research Program of Excellent Young Talents in Colleges and Universities of Anhui Provincial Education Department (GXGNFX2019120).

Conflict of interest

The authors declare no conflict of interest.

Author details

Qingqiang Lin[1], Hong Zhang[1], Jiuhua Zhao[2] and Zhengchao Wang[1*]

1 Provincial Key Laboratory for Developmental Biology and Neurosciences, College of Life Sciences, Fujian Normal University, Fuzhou, China

2 West Anhui Health Vocational College, Liuan, China

*Address all correspondence to: zcwang@fjnu.edu.cn

References

[1] March WA, Moore VM, Willson KJ, Phillips DI, Norman RJ, Davies MJ. The prevalence of polycystic ovary syndrome in a community sample assessed under contrasting diagnostic criteria. Human Reproduction. 2010;**25**(2):544-551. DOI: 10.1093/humrep/dep399

[2] Burghen GA, Givens JR, Kitabchi AE. Correlation of hyperandrogenism with hyperinsulinism in polycystic ovarian disease. The Journal of Clinical Endocrinology and Metabolism. 1980;**50**(1):113-116

[3] Macut D, Bjekić-Macut J, Rahelić D, Doknić M. Insulin and the polycystic ovary syndrome. Diabetes Research and Clinical Practice. 2017;**130**:163-170. DOI: 10.1016/j.diabres.2017.06.011

[4] Li Y, Chen C, Ma Y, Xiao J, Luo G, Li Y, et al. Multi-system reproductive metabolic disorder: Significance for the pathogenesis and therapy of polycystic ovary syndrome (PCOS). Life Sciences. 2019;**228**:167-175. DOI: 10.1016/j.lfs.2019.04.046

[5] Wikiera B, Zubkiewicz-Kucharska A, Nocoń-Bohusz J, Noczyńska A. Metabolic disorders in polycystic ovary syndrome. Pediatric Endocrinology, Diabetes, and Metabolism. 2017;**23**(4):204-208. DOI: 10.18544/PEDM-23.04.0094

[6] Glueck CJ, Goldenberg N. Characteristics of obesity in polycystic ovary syndrome: Etiology, treatment, and genetics. Metabolism. 2019;**92**:108-120. DOI: 10.1016/j.metabol.2018.11.002

[7] Meier RK. Polycystic ovary syndrome. The Nursing Clinics of North America. 2018;**53**(3):407-420. DOI: 10.1016/j.cnur.2018.04.008

[8] Pasquali R. Metabolic syndrome in polycystic ovary syndrome. Frontiers of Hormone Research. 2018;**49**:114-130. DOI: 10.1159/000485995

[9] Escobar-Morreale HF. Polycystic ovary syndrome: Definition, aetiology, diagnosis and treatment. Nature Reviews. Endocrinology. 2018;**14**(5): 270-284. DOI: 10.1038/nrendo.2018.24

[10] Dunaif A. Hyperandrogenic anovulation (PCOS): A unique disorder of insulin action associated with an increased risk of non-insulin-dependent diabetes mellitus. The American Journal of Medicine. 1995;**98**(1A):33S-39S

[11] Dunaif A. Insulin resistance and the polycystic ovary syndrome: Mechanism and implications for pathogenesis. Endocrine Reviews. 1997;**18**(6):774-800

[12] Bachelot A. Polycystic ovarian syndrome: Clinical and biological diagnosis. Annales de Biologie Clinique (Paris). 2016;**74**(6):661-667

[13] Wang F, Wang S, Zhang Z, Lin Q, Liu Y, Xiao Y, et al. Defective insulin signaling and the protective effects of dimethyldiguanide during follicular development in the ovaries of polycystic ovary syndrome. Molecular Medicine Reports. 2017;**16**(6):8164-8170. DOI: 10.3892/mmr.2017.7678

[14] Wang F, Zhang ZH, Xiao KZ, Wang ZC. Roles of hypothalamic-pituitary-adrenal axis and hypothalamus-pituitary-ovary axis in the abnormal endocrine functions in patients with polycystic ovary syndrome. Zhongguo Yi Xue Ke Xue Yuan Xue Bao. 2017;**39**(5):699-704. DOI: 10.3881/j.issn.1000-503X.2017.05.017

[15] Wu YQ, Chen LY, Zhang ZH, Wang ZC. Effects of phosphatidylinositol-3 kinase/protein kinase b/bone morphogenetic protein-15 pathway on the follicular development in the mammalian ovary. Zhongguo Yi Xue Ke Xue Yuan Xue Bao. 2013;**35**(2):224-228. DOI: 10.3881/j.issn.1000-503X.2013.02.018

[16] Zhang Z, Yu D, Yin D, Wang Z. Activation of PI3K/mTOR signaling pathway contributes to induction of vascular endothelial growth factor by hCG in bovine developing luteal cells. Animal Reproduction Science. 2011;**125**(1-4):42-48. DOI: 10.1016/j.anireprosci.2011.03.002

[17] Crespo RP, Bachega TASS, Mendonça BB, Gomes LG. An update of genetic basis of PCOS pathogenesis. Archives of Endocrinology Metabolism. 2018;**62**(3):352-361. DOI: 10.20945/2359-3997000000049

[18] Dunaif A, Thomas A. Current concepts in the polycystic ovary syndrome. Annual Review of Medicine. 2001;**52**:401-419

[19] Bernard L, Christin-Maître S, Basille C, Chabbert-Buffet N. Insulin resistance and polycystic ovary syndrome. Gynécologie, Obstétrique & Fertilité. 2003;**31**(2):109-116

[20] Vollenweider P. Insulin resistant states and insulin signaling. Clinical Chemistry and Laboratory Medicine. 2003;**41**(9):1107-1119

[21] Yildiz BO, Chang W, Azziz R. Polycystic ovary syndrome and ovulation induction. Minerva Ginecologica. 2003;**55**(5):425-439

[22] Baillargeon JP, Nestler JE. Polycystic ovary syndrome: A syndrome of ovarian hypersensitivity to insulin? The Journal of Clinical Endocrinology and Metabolism. 2006;**91**(1):22-24

[23] Nelson-Degrave VL, Wickenheisser JK, Hendricks KL, Asano T, Fujishiro M, Legro RS, et al. Alterations in mitogen-activated protein kinase kinase and extracellular regulated kinase signaling in theca cells contribute to excessive androgen production in polycystic ovary syndrome. Molecular Endocrinology. 2005;**19**(2):379-390

[24] Chen L, Hu LM, Wang YF, Yang HY, Huang XY, Zhou W, et al. Effect of sodium aescinate treatment on PCOS rat model with insulin resistance. Bratislavské Lekárske Listy. 2017;**118**(4):223-227. DOI: 10.4149/BLL_2017_044

[25] Lan ZJ, Krause MS, Redding SD, Li X, Wu GZ, Zhou HX, et al. Selective deletion of Pten in theca-interstitial cells leads to androgen excess and ovarian dysfunction in mice. Molecular and Cellular Endocrinology. 2017;**444**:26-37. DOI: 10.1016/j.mce.2017.01.043

[26] Restuccia DF, Hynx D, Hemmings BA. Loss of PKBβ/Akt2 predisposes mice to ovarian cyst formation and increases the severity of polycystic ovary formation in vivo. Disease Models & Mechanisms. 2012;**5**(3):403-411. DOI: 10.1242/dmm.008136

[27] Sekar N, Veldhuis JD. Concerted transcriptional activation of the low density lipoprotein receptor gene by insulin and luteinizing hormone in cultured porcine granulosa-luteal cells: Possible convergence of protein kinase a, phosphatidylinositol 3-kinase, and mitogen-activated protein kinase signaling pathways. Endocrinology. 2001;**142**(7):2921-2928

[28] Franks S. Polycystic ovary syndrome in adolescents. International Journal of Obesity. 2008;**32**(7):1035-1041. DOI: 10.1038/ijo.2008.61

[29] Wang F, Zhang Z, Wang Z, Xiao K, Wang Q, Su J, et al. Expression and clinical significance of the HIF-1a/ET-2 signaling pathway during the development and treatment of polycystic ovary syndrome. Journal of Molecular Histology. 2015;**46**(2):173-181. DOI: 10.1007/s10735-015-9609-4

[30] Zhang J, Zhang Z, Wu Y, Chen L, Luo Q, Chen J, et al. Regulatory effect of hypoxia-inducible factor-1α

on hCG-stimulated endothelin-2 expression in granulosa cells from the PMSG-treated rat ovary. The Journal of Reproduction and Development. 2012;**58**(6):678-684

[31] Weiss NS, Kostova E, Nahuis M, Mol BWJ, van der Veen F, van Wely M. Gonadotrophins for ovulation induction in women with polycystic ovary syndrome. Cochrane Database of Systematic Reviews. 2019;**1**:CD010290. DOI: 10.1002/14651858.CD010290.pub3

[32] Sagvekar P, Dadachanji R, Patil K, Mukherjee S. Pathomechanisms of polycystic ovary syndrome: Multidimensional approaches. Frontiers in Bioscience (Elite Edition). 2018;**10**:384-422

[33] Polak K, Czyzyk A, Simoncini T, Meczekalski B. New markers of insulin resistance in polycystic ovary syndrome. Journal of Endocrinological Investigation. 2017;**40**(1):1-8. DOI: 10.1007/s40618-016-0523-8

[34] Dhindsa G, Bhatia R, Dhindsa M, Bhatia V. Insulin resistance, insulin sensitization and inflammation in polycystic ovarian syndrome. Journal of Postgraduate Medicine. 2004;**50**(2):140-144

Chapter 7

Roles of ncRNAs in Ovarian Dysfunction of Polycystic Ovary Syndrome

Junyong Han, Zhen Yu, Gang Chen and Fan Wang

Abstract

Polycystic ovary syndrome (PCOS) is a common endocrine disease in women of childbearing age. Many heterogeneous clinical manifestations of PCOS, including hyperandrogenism, obesity, insulin resistance, hirsutism, acne, chronic anovulation and infertility, seriously affected the quality of life of women worldwide and made it difficult to clearly demonstrate the specific pathophysiology. In recent years, large-scale studies have shown that non-coding RNAs (ncRNAs) play an important role in the regulation of ovarian functions, which did not have the ability to encode proteins and could regulate hormone synthesis and germ cell development, differentiation, and apoptosis by silencing transposable elements and regulating coding genes. A number of researches by whole transcriptome sequencing of polycystic ovaries (PCO) from PCOS patients or PCOS model animals found that the abnormal expressions of many ncRNAs were involved in the regulation of ovarian dysfunctions of PCOS, including the development of oocytes, the microenvironment of follicular fluid, and the proliferation, differentiation, and apoptosis of granulosa cells. The present review focused on the roles of ncRNAs in the PCO of PCOS, in order to provide a theoretical basis for further understanding of the molecular mechanisms of PCO formation in PCOS.

Keywords: ncRNAs, granule cell, oocyte, follicle fluid, polycystic ovary syndrome

1. Introduction

Polycystic ovary syndrome (PCOS) is an endocrine and reproductive disease in women that often occurs during the childbearing years [1]. PCOS is closely related to metabolic syndrome, and has become an increasingly serious public health problem worldwide, these patients have an increased risk of endometrial cancer, type 2 diabetes, and cardiovascular disease. The clinical characteristics of PCOS women show heterogeneity, include excessive androgen, infertility, obesity, anovulation, irregular menstruation, polycystic ovaries (PCO), hairy and recurrent miscarriage, insulin resistance and abnormal blood lipids [2].

Anovulatory infertility of PCOS patients accounts for more than 75%, and the spontaneous abortion rate of them in early pregnancy is 30–50% [3, 4]. Ovulation failure (such as ovulation or anovulation) is the main clinical features of PCOS. There are a large number of small follicles in the bilateral ovaries of PCOS patients, which can not grow into dominant follicle, suggesting the occurrence of follicular dysplasia [5]. The processes of ovarian follicular development and atresia are a complex and delicate. However, ovulatory dysfunction in PCOS women is related to various factors such as abnormalities in proliferation and apoptosis of granule cells (GCs) and in follicular development and atresia. As is well-known that GCs are involved in the normal development and maturation of follicles. Some studies have found that the proliferation rate of GCs in PCOS patients is significantly higher, and the apoptotic rate is significantly lower [6, 7] suggesting that abnormalities in the proliferation and apoptosis of GCs may be a pathogenic mechanism of ovarian dysfunction of PCOS.

Due to the complexity of the etiology of PCOS, its specific pathophysiology has not yet been fully elucidated. More and more researches are currently being conducted to analyze the gene expression profiling of PCOS at the mRNA and protein levels, in order to explore its molecular mechanisms. PCOS is caused by the imbalance of multiple gene pathways [8]. The candidate genes are involved in sex hormone synthesis, insulin synthesis, chronic inflammatory factors, lipid metabolism, cell proliferation and apoptosis [8]. With the advancement of RNA sequencing technologies, many researchers have discovered that non-coding RNA (ncRNA, which refers to a class of RNA without open reading frame and can not translate into proteins) is involved in the regulation of numerous cell signaling pathways and biological processes for life activities, such as cell development, differentiation, apoptosis and hormone synthesis, and the occurrence and development of diseases [9].

Most of the human genome is transcribed into various ncRNAs, MicroRNA (miRNA) and long-chain non-coding RNAs (lncRNA) are hotspots for studying novel biomarkers and therapeutic targets in related diseases in recent years, such as cancer [10], diabetes [11] and PCOS [9]. Recent studies have shown that both miRNA and lncRNA play an important role in the pathogenesis of PCOS [9, 12]. miRNA and lncRNA can directly or indirectly affect the normal physiological functions of the ovaries, include the growth and development of follicles and oocytes [9, 12]. Moreover, ovarian dysfunction in PCOS seriously affects the reproductive capacity in reproductive women, but its specific molecular mechanism is not yet known. This chapter focuses on the roles of several ncRNAs in PCOS ovaries in recent years, which will help to further elucidate its pathogenesis and to discover new therapeutic targets.

2. ncRNA

ncRNAs as enzyme, regulatory signal, molecular sink, ligand, organizer of cellular structures, potential hormone and scaffold of molecular interactions, can play an important role in cell physiology and abnormal biological processes, such as nuclear transport, transcriptional regulation of genes, protein degradation, genomic imprinting and X chromosome silencing [13].

2.1 miRNAs

miRNAs are 21–23 nucleotides in length and widely found in eukaryotes, which can predict post-transcriptional regulation of at least half of the human transcriptome [14–16]. Mature miRNA is formed by removing and processing a longer primary transcript through a series of nucleases [17–19]. The main function of miRNAs is silencing or degrading the expressions of target genes at the post-transcriptional level by forming an RNA-induced silencing complex [20]. Abnormal expressions of miRNAs are associated with insulin resistance [21, 22], diabetes [11, 22, 23], inflammation [20, 23] and various cancer formations [10]. The expression profiles of some miRNAs in ovarian various cells and follicular fluids of PCOS patients exist significant differences, which had been involved in the occurrence and development of PCOS by affecting the post-transcriptional regulation of the target genesw [9, 12, 24].

2.2 lncRNAs

lncRNAs are a class of non-coding RNAs transcripts longer than 200 nucleotides in length, which produced by 4–9% of the sequence in mammalian genome [25, 26]. lncRNAs play critical roles in various human biological processes, such as chromatin modification, cell differentiation, proliferation and apoptosis, translational and post-translational regulation. Moreover, the abnormally expressed lncRNAs are involved in the occurrence and development of a variety of human diseases [27]. In recent years, more and more evidence has shown that lncRNAs are abnormally expressed in ovarian cumulus cells and/or GCs of PCOS patients [9, 28, 29]. These lncRNAs may be involved in ovarian steroid production, steroid receptor activity and IR, and future affect ovarian cell development, proliferation and apoptosis, which in turn leads to the occurrence of ovarian dysfunction of PCOS [28, 29].

3. PCO

PCO is one of the diagnostic indicators and symptoms for PCOS, which imaged the ovaries with ultrasound showing ≥12 follicles (each follicle is 2–9 mm in diameter) on one or both sides, and/or an ovarian volume ≥10 ml [5]. During the development and maturation of ovarian follicles, the oocyte interconnected and interdependent with surrounding GCs. The development of an oocyte requires GCs to provide nutrients, corresponding hormones and growth regulators [30, 31]. Abnormal interactions between GCs and oocytes are a possible cause of ovarian follicular dysplasia in PCOS [32]. Some vitro fertilization studies found that PCOS patients have a lower rate of implantation than normal women [33–35]. Microarray analysis indicated that abnormal endocrine and metabolism affect gene expression of oocytes in PCOS ovaries [36].

Moreover, ovarian follicular fluid is a fluid that fills the follicular cavity and surrounds cumulus cells. Follicular fluid is rich in substances such as hormones, growth factors, anti-apoptotic antibodies, various proteins, peptides, amino acids and nucleotides. Studies have confirmed that these substances are closely related to female reproductive system diseases, embryo quality and in vitro fertilization outcomes [37]. Therefore, the homeostasis of the microenvironment of follicular fluid directly affects follicular development and oocytes quality.

It is well known that insulin resistance and hyperinsulinemia play an important role in the pathophysiology of PCOS. Studies have found that most of PCOS patients with varying degrees of IR and compensatory hyperinsulinemia, including ovarian IR [38]. Ovarian GCs in PCOS patients are impaired by insulin-dependent glucose metabolism [38, 39]. Damaged glucose metabolism reduces the energy supply to GCs and oocytes, and thus hinders the proliferation of GCs and the development of oocytes [38, 39]. Therefore, GCs dysfunction is contributed to abnormal ovarian function in PCOS, including anovulation. Moreover, excessive apoptosis of cumulus GCs directly causes follicular dysplasia in PCOS, which are correlated with changes in ncRNAs expression profiles in follicular fluid. The abnormal expressions of ncRNAs from the ovaries of PCOS may contribute to its occurrence and development [9, 12, 40].

4. Effects of ncRNAs on ovarian dysfunction of PCOS

With the development of RNA sequencing technologies, many researchers have carried out miRNA or lncRNA sequencing studies on the ovaries of PCOS, in order to detect the molecular mechanisms of ovarian dysfunction. Studies have shown that compared with control rats, there are 129 miRNAs (49 miRNAs are up-regulated, 80 miRNAs are down-regulated) and 158 lncRNAs (114 lncRNAs are up-regulated, 44 lncRNAs are down-regulated) by deep-sequencing of ovaries tissue from letrozole-induced PCOS rats [41, 42]. Gene ontology (GO) and Kyoto encyclopedia of genes and genomes (KEG) Genes pathway analyzed and predicted that the differentially expressed ncRNAs in PCOS ovaries may be associated with abnormal ovarian GCs proliferation, apoptosis and steroidogenesis and ovarian insulin resistance [41, 42].

4.1 Roles of ncRNAs in the proliferation and apoptosis of GCs

4.1.1 miR-141-3p

In the ovaries of PCOS rat model, the expression of miR-141-3p is significantly decreased, which can target to death-associated protein kinase 1 (DAPK1) and mitogen-activated protein kinase 1 (MAPK1) signaling pathway to inhibit apoptosis of GCs, or regulate mitochondria-mediated apoptosis through phosphatidylinositol 3 kinase/protein kinase B (PI3K/Akt) and extracellular protein kinase (ERK) signaling pathways, and thus suppressing cell growth, promoting cell apoptosis, and further leading to the development of PCOS [41].

4.1.2 miR-483-5p

miR-483-5p is the most abundant known miRNA in human ovarian follicular fluid [43]. miR-483-5p is highly expressed in cumulus granulosa cells and follicular fluid of PCOS patients [44]. In PCOS cumulus cells, high concentrations of miR-483-5p hinders the expressions of Notch3 and MAPK3 protein by binding to the 3′UTR terminus of their mRNA, thereby blocking the Notch signaling pathway and the MAPK signaling pathway (the two pathways play an important role in cell proliferation, differentiation and apoptosis), which inhibits the proliferation and differentiation of cumulus GCs and promoted the apoptosis of GCs [44].

4.1.3 LncRNA CD36-005

lncRNA CD36-005 is a transcript encoding the fatty acid transporter CD36 gene, which may be involved in cell growth, development, transport, and metabolism by bioinformatics analysis [42, 45]. lncRNA CD36-005 is expressed in rat ovaries, and its expression level is related to the estrous cycle, which indicates that it plays a role in animal reproductive activities [45]. Moreover, the study found that lncRNA CD36-005 and CD36 were highly expressed in the ovaries of PCOS rats by high-throughput sequencing and qRT-PCR verification. lncRNA CD36-005 significantly inhibits the proliferation of GCs by reducing the viability and the S phase of the cell cycle, which may be involved in the pathogenesis of PCOS [42].

4.2 Roles of ncRNAs in ovarian steroidogenesis

4.2.1 miR-320

miR-320 is closely related to PCOS, especially in the process of follicular development [46, 47]. miR-320 can regulate the translation of its target genes by post-transcriptional regulation, thereby improving the levels of steroid hormones. miR-320 was down-regulated in cumulus GCs from PCOS ovaries [48], and its expression in follicular fluid was controversial [49]. miR-320 deficiency not only impairs the expression of the steroid synthase CYP11A1 and CYP19A1, but also enhances the steroidogenesis in CGs by directly regulating the RUNX2/CYP11AI cascade in the 3′UTR of Runx2, indicating that the cascade are a possible mechanism for the lack of estrogen synthesis in GCs of PCOS patients. In addition, miR-320 can target transcriptional factors E2F1 and steroidogenic factor-1 (SF-1) to inhibit the proliferation of GCs, and promote the synthesis of testosterone and progesterone [47].

4.2.2 LncRNA HCG26

lncRNA HCG26 is mainly distributed in the nucleus of ovarian GCs, which is highly expressed in PCOS patients [29]. HCG26 knockout can promote aromatase gene expression and estradiol synthesis, but can not affect the levels of androstenedione and follicle stimulating hormone, suggesting lncRNA HCG26 is involved in abnormal ovarian steroidogenic synthesis [50]. Moreover, the study also found that lncRNA HCG26 deficiency inhibits the proliferation of GCs and its expression correlated with the number of PCOS ovarian follicles, suggesting that lncRNA HCG26 may affect the proliferation of GCs and contributes to the formation of polycystic ovary morphology [29].

4.3 Roles of ncRNAs in ovarian insulin resistance

4.3.1 miR-92

Down-regulation of miR-92a/b expression in PCOS patients is associated with insulin resistance, hyperinsulinemia and hyperandrogenism [24], which can increase the expression of its target gene IRS-2, which activates the insulin signaling pathway in the ovaries of PCOS patients, thereby leading to be involved in the process of insulin resistance and hyperinsulinemia [24, 29].

4.3.2 miR-145

miR-145 overexpression in GCs of PCOS patients inhibits the target gene IRS1 and MAPK/ERK signaling pathways, and promotes the activity of PI3K/Akt signaling pathway through negative feedback, thereby improving IR in PCOS patients [7, 24, 50].

5. Conclusions

PCOS is a chronic disease that affects the patients throughout their lives. However, there is currently no gene that is recognized as the determinant of the pathogenesis of PCOS. Although the differential expression of ncRNAs in the ovaries from PCOS are involving in ovarian steroidogenesis, insulin resistance, cell proliferation and apoptosis and affect follicular development by regulating the expression of corresponding target genes at the post-transcriptional level, there are still many ncRNAs and the specific mechanism of their action in ovarian function of PCOS have not been discovered. Moreover, the roles and mechanisms of lncRNAs in PCOS have just been carried out, and the focus is on the study of lncRNA in peripheral blood of the patients or animal models, that in ovarian tissue is limited. The interactions between ncRNAs in PCOS have not been reported, such as miRNA-miRNA, lncRNA-lncRNA, and miRNA-lncRNA. Solving these problems will be contribution to further understand the etiology and pathogenesis of PCOS.

Acknowledgements

This study was supported by Young and Middle-aged Talents Training Project of Fujian Provincial Health and Family Planning (2018-ZQN-20).

Conflict of interest

The authors declare no conflict of interest.

A. Appendices

PCOS	polycystic ovary syndrome
ncRNAs	non-coding RNA
PCO	polycystic ovary
GCs	granule cells
lncRNA	long-chain non-coding RNAs
GO	gene ontology
KEGG	Kyoto encyclopedia of genes and genomes
DAPK1	death-associated protein kinase 1
MAP K1	mitogen-activated protein kinase 1
PI3K/Akt	phosphatidylinositol 3 kinase/protein kinase B
ERK	extracellular protein kinase
SF-1	steroidogenic factor-1

Author details

Junyong Han[1], Zhen Yu[1], Gang Chen[1] and Fan Wang[1,2,3]*

1 Fujian Provincial Key Laboratory of Medical Analysis, Fujian Academy of Medical Sciences, Fuzhou, China

2 State Key Laboratory for Evaluation of Exercise Physiological Functions from General Administration of Sport of China, School of Physical Education and Sport Sciences, Fujian Normal University, Fuzhou, China

3 Laboratory of Sport Physiology and Biomedicine, School of Physical Education and Sport Sciences, Fujian Normal University, Fuzhou, China

*Address all correspondence to: 517239819@qq.com

References

[1] Bazarganipour F, Taghavi SA, Montazeri A, Ahmadi F, Chaman R, Khosravi A. The impact of polycystic ovary syndrome on the health-related quality of life: A systematic review and meta-analysis. International Journal of Reproductive Biomedicine. 2015;**13**(2):61-70

[2] Fan W, Shaobing W, Zhenghong Z, Qingqiang L, Yiping L, Yijun X, et al. Defective insulin signaling and the protective effects of dimethyldiguanide during follicular development in the ovaries of polycystic ovary syndrome. Molecular Medicine Reports. 2017;**16**(6):8164-8170. DOI: 10.3892/mmr.2017.7678

[3] Caldwell A, Edwards M, Desai R, Jimenez M, Gilchrist RB, Handelsman DJ, et al. Neuroendocrine androgen action is a key extraovarian mediator in the development of polycystic ovary syndrome. Proceedings of the National Academy of Sciences of the United States of America. 2017;**114**(16):E3334-E3343. DOI: 10.1073/pnas.1616467114

[4] Xuezhou Y, Xiaozhen Q, Yanli L, Qipeng W, Jinhai Y, Xiaofang Y, et al. Serum chemerin level in women with PCOS and its relation with the risk of spontaneous abortion. Gynecological Endocrinology. 2018;**34**(10):864-867. DOI: 10.1080/09513590.2018.1462316

[5] Giampaolino P, Della Corte L, De Rosa N, Mercorio A, Bruzzese D, Bifulco G. Ovarian volume and PCOS: A controversial issue. Gynecological Endocrinology. 2018;**34**(3):229-232. DOI: 10.1080/09513590.2017.1391205

[6] Song WJ1, Shi X, Zhang J, Chen L, Fu SX, Ding YL. Akt-mTOR signaling mediates abnormalities in the proliferation and apoptosis of ovarian granulosa cells in patients with polycystic ovary syndrome. Gynecologic and Obstetric Investigation. 2018;**83**(2):124-132. DOI: 10.1159/000464351

[7] Cai G, Ma X, Chen B, Huang Y, Liu S, Yang H, et al. MicroRNA-145 negatively regulates cell proliferation through targeting IRS1 in isolated ovarian granulosa cells from patients with polycystic ovary syndrome. Reproductive Sciences. 2016;**24**(6):902-910. DOI: 10.1177/1933719116673197

[8] Li L, Baek KH. Molecular genetics of polycystic ovary syndrome: An update. Current Molecular Medicine. 2015;**15**(4):331-342. DOI: 10.2174/1566524015666150505160140

[9] Qian Y, Chengliang Z, Jiexue P, Huanghe F. Research advances in the roles of ncRNAs in polycystic ovary syndrome. Journal of Shanghai Jiaotong University. 2016;**36**(6):921-925. DOI: 10.3969/j.issn.1674-8115.2016.06.027

[10] Trang P, Weidhaas JB, Slack FJ. MicroRNAs and cancer. In: Coleman W, Tsongalis G, editors. The Molecular Basis of Human Cancer. New York, NY: Humana Press; 2017. https://doi.org/10.1007/978-1-59745-458-2_17

[11] Tian Y, Xu J, Du X, Fu X. The interplay between noncoding RNAs and insulin in diabetes. Cancer Letters. 2018;**419**:53-63. DOI: 10.1016/j.canlet.2018.01.038

[12] Huang X, Liu C, Hao C, Tang Q, Liu R, Lin S, et al. Identification of altered microRNAs and mRNAs in the cumulus cells of PCOS patients. Reproduction. 2016;**151**(6):643-655. DOI: 10.1530/REP-16-0071

[13] Fu XD. Non-coding RNA: A new frontier in regulatory biology. National Science Review. 2014;**1**(2):190-204. DOI: 10.1093/nsr/nwu008

[14] Yanli W, Meiling Y, En-Bo M, Jianzhen Z. Identification and analysis of the miRNAs targeting key genes involved in cuticle metabolism in Locusta migratoria (orthoptera:Acrididae). Acta Entomologica Sinica. 2017;**60**(3):309-317. DOI: 10.16380/j.kcxb.2017.03.008

[15] Davis-Dusenbery BN, Hata A. Mechanisms of control of microRNA biogenesis. Journal of Biochemistry. 2010;**148**(4):381-392. DOI: 10.1093/jb/mvq096

[16] Jinbiao M, Ying H. Post-transcriptional regulation of miRNA biogenesis and functions. Frontiers in Biology. 2010;**5**(1):32-40. DOI: 10.1007/s11515-010-0004-y

[17] Büssing I, Yang JS, Lai EC, Grosshans H. The nuclear export receptor XPO-1 supports primary miRNA processing in C. elegans and drosophila. EMBO Journal. 2014;**29**(11):1830-1839. DOI: 10.1038/emboj.2010.82

[18] Kawahara H, Imai T, Okano H. MicroRNAs in neural stem cells and neurogenesis. Frontiers in Neuroscience. 2012;**6**:30. DOI: 10.3389/fnins.2012.00030

[19] Wu K, He J, Pu W, Yong P. The role of exportin-5 in MicroRNA biogenesis and cancer. Genomics, Proteomics & Bioinformatics. 2018;**65**(5):42-46. DOI: 10.1016/j.gpb.2017.09.004

[20] Singh RP, Massachi I, Manickavel S, Singh S, Rao NP, Hasan S, et al. The role of miRNA in inflammation and autoimmunity. Autoimmunity Reviews. 2013;**12**(12):1160-1165. DOI: 10.1016/j.autrev.2013.07.003

[21] Williams MD, Mitchell GM. MicroRNAs in insulin resistance and obesity. Experimental Diabetes Research. 2015;**2012**(3):484696. DOI: 10.1155/2012/484696

[22] Honardoost M, Sarookhani MR, Arefian E, Soleimani M. Insulin resistance associated genes and miRNAs. Applied Biochemistry and Biotechnology. 2014;**174**(1):63-80. DOI: 10.1007/s12010-014-1014-z

[23] Leti F, Taila M, Distefano JK. The role of ncRNA in diabetes[M]. In: MicroRNAs and Other Non-Coding RNAs in Inflammation. 2015

[24] Saihua Z, Xuelian L, Gynecology DO. Expression and effect of MicroRNA in patients with polycystic ovary syndrome. International Journal of Reproductive Health/Family Planning. 2016;**35**(2):146-150

[25] Qi P, Xiaoyan Z, Xiang D. Circulating long non-coding RNAs in cancer: Current status and future perspectives. Molecular Cancer. 2016;**15**(1):39. DOI: 10.1186/s12943-016-0524-4

[26] Zhiping Z, Jian L, Yunchao W, Huan Q, Weiwu G, Chenhui W, et al. Effect of LncRNA LOC100506123 on proliferation and migration in pancreatic cancer cells. Journal of Third Military Medical University. 2017;**39**(9):840-845. DOI: 10.16016/j.1000-5404.201611074

[27] Ping P, Wang L, Kuang L, Ye S, MFB I, Pei T. A novel method for LncRNA-disease association prediction based on an lncRNA-disease association network. IEEE/ACM Transactions on Computational Biology and Bioinformatics. 2019;**16**(2):688-693. DOI: 10.1109/TCBB.2018.2827373

[28] Xin H, Cuifang H, Hongchu B, Meimei W, Huangguan D. Aberrant expression of long noncoding RNAs in cumulus cells isolated from PCOS patients. Journal of Assisted Reproduction and Genetics. 2016;**33**(1):111-121. DOI: 10.1007/s10815-015-0630-z

[29] Yudong L, Ying L, Shuxian F, Desheng Y, Xin C, Xingyu Z, et al. Long noncoding RNAs: Potential regulators involved in the pathogenesis of polycystic ovary syndrome. Endocrinology. 2017;**158**(11):3890-3899. DOI: 10.1210/en.2017-00605

[30] Munakata Y, Ichinose T, Ogawa K, tami N, Tasaki H, Shirasuna K, et al. Relationship between the number of cells surrounding oocytes and energy states of oocytes. Theriogenology. 2016;**86**(7):1789-1798.e1. DOI: 10.1016/j.theriogenology.2016.05.036

[31] Zhengbin H, Guocheng L, Yanguang W, Dong H, Weiguo F, Junzuo W, et al. Interactive effects of granulosa cell apoptosis, follicle size, cumulus-oocyte complex morphology, and cumulus expansion on the developmental competence of goat oocytes: A study using the well-in-drop culture system. Reproduction. 2006;**132**(5):749-758. DOI: 10.1530/REP-06-0055

[32] Kim E, Seok HH, Lee SY, Lee DR, Moon J, Yoon TK, et al. Correlation between expression of glucose transporters in granulosa cells and oocyte quality in women with polycystic ovary syndrome. Endocrinology & Metabolism. 2014;**29**(1):40-47. DOI: 10.3803/EnM.2014.29.1.40

[33] Ashkenazi J, Farhi J, Orvieto R, Homburg R, Dekel A, Feldberg D, et al. Polycystic ovary syndrome patients as oocyte donors: The effect of ovarian stimulation protocol on the implantation rate of the recipient. Fertility and Sterility. 1995;**64**(3):564-567. DOI: 10.1016/s0015-0282(16)57793-0

[34] Jabara S, Coutifaris C. In vitro fertilization in the PCOS patient: Clinical considerations. Seminars in Reproductive Medicine. 2003;**21**(03):317-324. DOI: 10.1055/s-2003-43310

[35] Li R, Qiao J. The different endometrial receptivity between the normal women and PCOS patients in the implantation window. Chinese Journal of Birth Health & Heredity. 2007;**84**(3):S456-S456. DOI: 10.1016/j.fertnstert.2005.07.1193

[36] Wood JR, Dumesic DA, Abbott DH, Strauss JF. Molecular abnormalities in oocytes from women with polycystic ovary syndrome revealed by microarray analysis. The Journal of Clinical Endocrinology and Metabolism. 2007;**92**(2):705-713. DOI: 10.1210/jc.2006-2123

[37] Klein NA, Battaglia DE, Miller PB, Branigan EF, Giudice LC, Soules MR. Ovarian follicular development and the follicular fluid hormones and growth factors in normal women of advanced reproductive age. The Journal of Clinical Endocrinology & Metabolism. 1996;**81**(5):1946-1951. DOI: 10.1210/jcem.81.5.8626862

[38] Ciaraldi TP. Molecular defects of insulin action in the polycystic ovary syndrome: Possible tissue specificity. Journal of Pediatric Endocrinology & Metabolism. 2000;**13**(Suppl 5):1291 1293. DOI: 10.1046/j.1440-1754.2000.00616.x

[39] Diamanti-Kandarakis E, Argyrakopoulou G, Economou F, Kandaraki E, Koutsilieris M. Defects in insulin signaling pathways in ovarian steroidogenesis and other tissues in polycystic ovary syndrome (PCOS). The Journal of Steroid Biochemistry and Molecular Biology. 2008;**109**(3-5):242-246. DOI: 10.1016/j.jsbmb.2008.03.014

[40] Xiaoke W, Risto E. Ovarian insulin resistance and insulin sensitizer effect on polycystic ovary syndrome. Zhonghua Fu Chan Ke Za Zhi. 2005;**39**(12):804-808. DOI: http://dx.DOI.org/

[41] Li D, Xu D, Xu Y, Chen L, Li C, Dai X, et al. MicroRNA-141-3p

targets DAPK1 and inhibits apoptosis in rat ovarian granulosa cells. Cell Biochemistry and Function. 2017;**35**:197-201. DOI: 10.1002/cbf.3248

[42] Lulu F, Ying X, Dandan L, Xiaowei D, Xin X, Jingshun Z, et al. Expression profiles of mRNA and long noncoding RNA in the ovaries of letrozole-induced polycystic ovary syndrome rat model through deep sequencing. Gene. 2018;**657**:19-29. DOI: 10.1016/j.gene.2018.03.002

[43] Hua X, Xiaoyan Y, Boqun X. Involvement of MiRNA in pathogenesis of polycystic ovary syndrome. International Journal of Reproductive Health/Family Planning. 2017;**1**:66-69. DOI: 10.3969/j.issn.1674-1889.2017.01.018

[44] B Xu, YW Zhang, XH Tong, YS Liu. Characterization of microRNA profile in human cumulus granulosa cells: Identification of microRNAs that regulate notch signaling and are associated with PCOS. Molecular and Cellular Endocrinology. 2015;**404**:26-36. DOI: 10.1016/j.mce.2015.01.030

[45] Xueying Z, Ying X, Lulu F, Dandan L. Identification of mRNAs related to endometrium function regulated by lncRNA CD36-005 in rat endometrial stromal cells. Reproductive Biology and Endocrinology. 2018;**16**(1):96. DOI: 10.1186/s12958-018-0412-4

[46] Ruizhi F, Qing S, Yan Z, Wei F, Miao L, Yan X, et al. MiRNA-320 in the human follicular fluid is associated with embryo quality in vivo and affects mouse embryonic development in vitro. Scientific Reports. 2015;**5**:8689. DOI: 10.1038/srep08689

[47] Mianmian Y, Xiaorong W, Guidong Y, Mingrong L, Meng L, Yingpu S, et al. Transactivation of miR-320 by miR-383 regulates granulosa cell functions by targeting E2F1 and SF-1. Journal of Biological Chemistry. 2014;**289**(26):18239-18257. DOI: 10.1074/jbc.M113.546044

[48] Chenling Z, Hui W, Changyou Y, Xuefeng G, Xiaojuan L. Deregulation of RUNX2 by miR-320a deficiency impairs steroidogenesis in cumulus granulosa cells from polycystic ovary syndrome (PCOS) patients. Biochemical and Biophysical Research Communications. 2017;**482**(4):1469-1476. DOI: 10.1016/j.bbrc.2016.12.059

[49] SørensenRensen A, Louise Wissing M, Salö S, Lis Mikkelsen Englund A. MicroRNAs related to polycystic ovary syndrome (PCOS). Genes. 2014;**5**(3):684-708. DOI: 10.3390/genes5030684

[50] Naji M, Nekoonam S, Aleyasin A, Arefian E, Mahdian R, Azizi E, et al. Expression of miR-15a, miR-145, and miR-182 in granulosa-lutein cells, follicular fluid, and serum of women with polycystic ovary syndrome (PCOS). Archives of Gynecology and Obstetrics. 2017;**297**(1):221-231. DOI: 10.1007/s00404-017-4570-y

Chapter 8

Interplay between Oxidative Stress and Chronic Inflammation in PCOS: The Role of Genetic Variability in PCOS Risk and Treatment Responses

Rok Herman, Mojca Jensterle Sever, Andrej Janež and Vita Dolžan

Abstract

PCOS is often accompanied by insulin resistance, which is associated with the pathogenesis of the syndrome and increases the risk of developing the metabolic syndrome, type 2 diabetes, and cardiovascular complications. All these processes are characterized by chronic inflammation, which may be associated with an increased formation of reactive oxygen species and activation of inflammatory pathways that may further aggravate the function of pancreatic beta-cells. It has been shown that PCOS treatment improves metabolic indexes, while at the same time lowering inflammatory indicators. This chapter summarizes the latest findings about the role of oxidative stress and chronic inflammation in pathogenesis of PCOS. It also provides information on genetic variability in these pathways that may lead to interindividual differences in the risk for PCOS-related metabolic complications. Furthermore, genetic variability in these pathways may influence response to different treatment options in PCOS patients.

Keywords: PCOS, insulin resistance, chronic inflammation, oxidative stress, reactive oxygen species, inflammatory pathways, metabolic syndrome

1. Introduction

Polycystic ovarian syndrome (PCOS) is the most common endocrine disorder in women in the reproductive period as it affects between 4 and 12% of the female population. Nowadays, it is known that both genetic and environmental factors play a role in PCOS development and its numerous clinical manifestations. The syndrome is characterized by hyperandrogenism, ovarian dysfunction and polycystic ovaries, insulin resistance (IR), and chronic inflammation, all of which in the long term also affects the post-reproductive period. It is associated with the increased risk for infertility, depression, cardiovascular diseases (CVD), and endometrial and even breast cancer [1].

PCOS develops, when ovaries produce an excessive amount of male sex hormones, androgens, in particular, testosterone and androstenedione. This occurs due to two main reasons. The first one is irregular pulsative secretion of luteinizing hormone (LH) from the adenohypophysis, which then increases the production of androgens. The second mechanism is more complex, and it involves IR with associated increased concentration of serum insulin. Insulin stimulates pathways that activate ovarian androgen production while at the same time lowering serum sex hormone-binding globulin (SHBG) concentrations. Patients also intrinsically have higher serum levels of gonadotropin-releasing hormone, which increases the ratio between the LH and follicle-stimulating hormone (FSH). Higher ratio leads to increased androgen production, slower follicle maturation, and decreased binding of sex hormones on SHBG [2].

The choice of treatment is influenced by the desired goals, which in most cases are the treatment for infertility and obesity and the reduction of symptoms of hyperandrogenism. Clomiphene and letrozole are first-line medications for infertility. If patients do not desire pregnancy, hormonal contraceptives are recommended for irregular menses and dermatologic manifestations. Metformin is the first-line treatment for metabolic manifestations. Glucagon-like peptide 1 (GLP-1)-based therapies and glitazones can be used in most severe cardio-metabolic PCOS phenotypes that are resistant to first-line treatments [3, 4].

For quite some time, the subject of research has also been the involvement of chronic inflammation and oxidative stress (OS) in the pathogenesis of PCOS. Several studies have already confirmed that patients have elevated levels of OS and inflammatory mediators and, on the other hand, have decreased antioxidant capacity. There is also an unanswered question of the extent to which OS and inflammation are causally related.

Research has already confirmed that genetic changes in key antioxidant enzymes and inflammatory mediators can affect the individual's defense ability against OS and their predisposition to inflammation. Nowadays, molecular genetic analysis is increasingly being used in clinical practice as it is a widely available method, easily accessible and inexpensive. It also enables identification of groups of patients with an increased risk of developing various diseases and offers a patient-adapted treatment, thereby representing one of the pillars of personalized medicine.

2. Chronic inflammation in PCOS

Inflammation is arguably involved to some degree in the underlying causes of many chronic diseases. It is well known that different types of inflammatory cytokines and chemokines are involved in female reproductive processes, including ovulation, follicular development, fertilization, implantation, and pregnancy [5]. While the exact etiology of PCOS still remains unknown, the amount of evidence in support of an important role of chronic low-grade inflammation in this process is increasing. Chronic proinflammatory state in women with this syndrome is also likely to be associated with other clinical manifestations and complications of PCOS, including IR and CVD.

When studying the relationship between PCOS and chronic inflammation, it is impossible to completely disregard the influence of increased body mass index (BMI) in patients with increased inflammation markers. Similar to PCOS, low-grade chronic inflammation is also present in metabolic syndrome (MS) [6]. This proinflammatory state may be an important part of the pathogenesis of both syndromes and one of the reasons why they often overlap. The relationship between them is mutual: PCOS women have a higher prevalence of MS, and alternatively, women with MS commonly present the reproductive and endocrine traits of PCOS. The visceral adipose tissue plays a key role in this overlap. It is more abundant and metabolically active in both syndromes, which results in an increased turnover of free fatty acids and an excessive secretion of several molecules, some of which are inflammatory markers [7]. There is still not enough evidence to conclude whether the proinflammatory state is intrinsic to PCOS, or it is rather only a consequence of higher amounts of dysfunctional adipose tissue in those patients. In favor of the latter theory are many studies which show that the higher the BMI in PCOS women, the greater the inflammatory state. However, the fact that PCOS women with lower BMI have more inflammation than healthy controls with higher BMI indicates that chronic low-grade inflammation may not be dependent on increased body mass only [8].

We can find the same degree of uncertainty in the relationship between chronic inflammation and excessive androgen secretion in PCOS. It is unclear whether androgen excess in PCOS promotes proinflammatory state or conversely whether the inflammatory molecules stimulate ovarian androgen production and hyperandrogenemia. Androgens influence the expression of different proteins and enzymes in adipocytes and cause their hypertrophy. Also, hyperandrogenism in PCOS increases mononuclear cell sensitivity to ingested glucose and promotes activation of mononuclear cells. This leads to another important concept in PCOS: diet-induced inflammation. Studies have shown that glucose ingested in vivo, as well as glucose exposure in vitro, stimulates an inflammatory response by promoting the mononuclear cells to release tumor necrosis factor alpha (TNFα) and interleukin 6 (IL-6) [9]. Furthermore, infiltration of ovarian tissue by macrophages and increased concentrations of TNFα and IL-6 in the follicular fluid (FF) have been previously demonstrated in women with PCOS. It is possible to suspect that mononuclear cells recruited into the polycystic ovaries cause a local inflammatory response that stimulates CYP17, the ovarian steroidogenic enzyme, responsible for androgen production. This establishes the vicious cycle, which indicates that inflammation alone can promote androgen secretion, and this androgen excess can stimulate inflammation through adipocyte hypertrophy and increased mononuclear cell sensitivity to ingested glucose [9].

One of the most often used inflammatory markers is C-reactive protein (CRP). It is primarily synthesized by the liver as an acute-phase protein. There is now growing evidence that CRP has important roles in inflammatory pathways and host responses to infection including the complement pathway, apoptosis, phagocytosis, nitric oxide (NO) release, and the production of cytokines, particularly IL-6 and TNFα [10]. The first study which demonstrated elevation of serum CRP concentrations in women with PCOS was carried out by Kelly and associates in 2001. They compared 17 women with PCOS and 15 healthy women and concluded that women with PCOS had significantly increased CRP concentrations relative to women with normal menstrual rhythm and normal androgen levels. They were also one of the first to propose low-grade chronic inflammation as a novel mechanism contributing to increased risk of CVD and type 2 diabetes in these women [11]. These findings paved the way for numerous further studies. The first big meta-analysis of all these studies was conducted in 2011 and included 3.648 women in total, and among them, 2.359 had PCOS and 1.289 were healthy controls. Mean serum CRP levels were 95% higher in women with PCOS than controls. Elevated circulating CRP levels in PCOS women were independent of obesity because the finding persisted after excluding all the studies with mismatches in the frequency of obesity or body mass between groups from the meta-analysis [8]. Some studies examined the effects of different treatment options on CRP levels. Metformin was shown to significantly lower the CRP levels in different treatment protocols [12, 13]. Recent studies also noticed that other PCOS management options, like statins or even increased physical activity only, significantly decreased CRP levels in women with PCOS [14, 15].

When considering other traditional inflammatory markers, females with PCOS were reported to have significantly higher levels of serum monocytes, lymphocytes, eosinophilic granulocytes, TNFα, and IL-6 than controls. Besides, in PCOS, ovarian tissue has more macrophages and lymphocytes than controls. Lymphocytes and macrophages secrete inflammatory cytokines like TNFα and IL-6, which in turn activate more lymphocytes and macrophages to enhance further cytokine secretion [9]. Especially TNFα seems to play a significant role in various clinical manifestations of PCOS. It is one of the most well-known inflammatory factors and has strong scientific evidence to be an important mediator in processes such as obesity, IR, and androgen expression. As a multifunctional hormone-like polypeptide, it has a wide variety of physiological roles including many directly connected with ovaries, such as regulation of ovarian function and exerting an influence on proliferation, differentiation, follicular maturation, steroidogenesis, and apoptosis [16]. A meta-analysis, published in 2016, which examined results from 29 studies with a total of 1960 women (1046 PCOS patients and 914 controls), concluded that TNFα levels in women with PCOS were significantly higher than healthy controls and that high-serum TNFα concentration was related to IR and androgen excess but not to the BMI [17]. TNFα is overexpressed in adipose tissue, so the source of excess circulating TNFα in PCOS is mostly adipose tissue in the obese but remains unknown in lean women with this disorder [18]. To even further emphasize the important role of TNFα in PCOS, its concentration is not elevated on a systemic level only but also in FF. Changes in FF levels of TNFα are associated with poor-quality oocytes in women undergoing in vitro fertilization, which then leads to a reduction in rates of fertilization, embryonic development, and pregnancy outcome [16]. Among other mechanisms, TNFα production is also induced by another proinflammatory cytokine interleukin 18 (IL-18), which was also reported to be increased in PCOS. It is produced by macrophages and induces cell-mediated immunity. Studies suggest that its levels are higher even in lean PCOS patients and are correlated with IR and CVD risk [19, 20].

TNFα promotes the synthesis of two other important cytokines, IL-6 and interleukin 8 (IL-8). IL-8 is mainly synthesized in macrophages and monocytes and is a significant immune response modulator. However, there are more studies regarding the role of IL-6 in PCOS, which has been closely associated with IR and CVD. Obesity was reported to be correlated with elevated IL-6 levels. In contrast, IL-6 levels decreased in PCOS patients after reducing their level of IR and body mass. Although some studies reported significant elevations in IL-6 levels in women with PCOS compared with controls, these findings were not confirmed in similar studies, with some studies even reporting decreased IL-6 levels in patients. However, a meta-analysis published in 2016, which included 922 PCOS patients and 696 controls, suggested that IL-6 levels were higher in women with PCOS than BMI-matched controls and that a high-serum IL-6 concentration was related to IR and androgen levels, but not to the BMI [21]. In a research article published in Mediators of Inflammation in 2011, authors concluded that IL-6 production and serum levels are related to an altered immune response in PCOS women with IR. They divided 44 young girls with PCOS aged 15–23 into non-IR and IR groups based on homeostatic model assessment (HOMA) findings. They were weight- and age-matched with healthy young girls, and they measured a variety of different inflammatory markers. The biggest difference between groups was in significant higher IL-6 levels in IR PCOS patients. Moreover, in the PCOS group, lipopolysaccharide-activated monocytes secreted significantly higher levels of IL-6 [22].

Several studies investigated two other important cytokines, interleukin 10 (IL-10) and interleukin 1 (IL-1) family in PCOS patients. The former is an important anti-inflammatory cytokine with multiple effects in immunoregulation and inflammation. In a study including 61 PCOS patients and 80 healthy controls, IL-10 levels were significantly lower among PCOS patients [23]. On the other hand, IL-1 family is a group of 11 cytokines that are primarily associated with innate immunity and are closely linked to a proinflammatory response. The IL-1 gene cluster on chromosome 2 contains three related genes *IL-1α*, *IL-1β*, and *IL-1RN*, encoding the proinflammatory cytokines IL-1α and IL-1β and their endogenous receptor antagonist. Previous PCOS research has been focused mainly on IL-1β since many studies suggested its crucial role in inflammatory-linked mechanisms in the ovaries. It probably intervenes in prostaglandin production, mainly by its activity on cyclooxygenase-2 synthesis. It also stimulates the production of other inflammatory cytokines, such as IL-6 and interleukin 12 (IL-12) [24].

At the beginning of this century, Jurg Tschopp introduced the concept of the inflammasome, and since then, inflammasomes have become an important topic of immunological studies. The inflammasome is a macromolecular cytoplasm complex that senses many different signals for cell damage on the molecular level and initiates the inflammatory response. It promotes the maturation and secretion of proinflammatory cytokines IL-1β, IL-18, and interferon gamma (IFNγ) and activates nuclear factor κB (NF-κB). There are many different types of inflammasomes, but NLRP3 inflammasome is most commonly associated with obesity and IR. It consists of three subunits: NLRP3, the adaptor protein apoptosis-associated speck-like protein (ASC), and caspase-1. It initiates an inflammatory form of cell death and triggers the release of proinflammatory cytokine IL-1β through the mechanism of procaspase-1 cleavage. However, the role of NLRP3 inflammasome in the development of PCOS remains largely unknown [25]. In a study published in 2017, the NLRP3 and ASC mRNA levels, caspase-1 activation, and IL-1β production were unregulated in PCOS patients, and those levels significantly improved after treatment with dimethylbiguanide [26]. NLRP3 inflammasome may present an important overlapping pathway between OS and chronic inflammation in PCOS, which will be discussed in further detail in Chapter 4. In contrast with other previously described inflammatory markers, there have been no published studies regarding different genetic polymorphisms in NLRP3 inflammasome and PCOS at the time of writing. However, there is a lot of evidence that gain-of-function polymorphisms in the NLRP3 inflammasome play an important role in rheumatoid arthritis and Crohn's disease [27].

There has been a lot of progress in the pharmacogenetics of PCOS in recent years. Its main goal is to find associations between genetic polymorphisms and the course of the disease and response to treatment. In **Table 1**, we summarized main studies which pointed out positive associations between different polymorphisms in genes related to previously described inflammatory markers and PCOS risk or clinical manifestations. At the time of writing, we could not find any study which would explore the relationship between polymorphisms in those genes and treatment response.

Gene	Variants	Predicted effect	Reference
TNFα	rs1799964 −1031 T > C	*Susceptibility* The TT genotype was more frequent in controls ($p = 0.0002$) and TC genotype in patients ($p = 0.0003$) *Clinical manifestations* TC genotype was associated with lower BMI ($p = 0.03$). TT genotype was associated with early onset and hyperandrogenism ($p < 0.05$)	[28]
		Susceptibility The frequency distribution of TT, TC, and CC genotypes differed between PCOS and control group ($p = 0.0003$)	[29]
		Susceptibility A significant difference in allele transmission was found in families with proband for PCOS ($p = 0.0013$)	[30]
	rs1799724 −857 C > T	*Susceptibility* T allele showed a protective role against PCOS ($p = 0.0032$)	[31]
	rs4645843 6213 C > T	*Susceptibility* Genotype and allele distribution differed significantly between PCOS patients and controls ($p = 0.03$ and 0.024, respectively) *Clinical manifestations* Polymorphism was significantly associated with serum testosterone levels ($p = 0.01$), HOMA-IR ($p = 0.034$), and BMI ($p < 0.05$).	[32]
IL-6	rs1800795 −174 G > C	*Susceptibility* Genotype and allele distribution differed significantly between PCOS patients and controls. The G allele frequency was significantly higher in PCOS patients than controls (all p values < 0.05)	[33]
		Susceptibility Polymorphism was associated with decreased PCOS susceptibility in the overall population under the allelic model (G vs. C, $p = 0.005$), the homozygous model (GG vs. CC, $p = 0.001$), heterozygous model (GG vs. CG, $p = 0.036$), and the dominant model (GC+CC vs. GG, $p = 0.020$)	[34]
		Susceptibility G allele was more frequent in patients with hyperandrogenism both when only homozygous and when homozygous and heterozygous G allele carriers were considered ($p < 0.05$ for all analyses)	[35]
		Susceptibility The genotype as well as the polymorphic G allele distribution differed between PCOS patients and controls (both $p < 0.001$)	[36]
		Clinical manifestations A relationship was detected between hirsutism, FSH, LH, total testosterone, HDL-cholesterol and triglyceride levels, and CG+GG genotypes. Furthermore, an association was found between IL-6 levels and CC genotype in the obese PCOS patients ($p < 0.05$ for all analyses)	[37]
	rs1800797 −597 A > G	*Susceptibility* G allele was more frequent in patients with hyperandrogenism both when only homozygous and when homozygous and heterozygous G allele carriers were considered ($p < 0.05$ for all analyses)	[35]

Gene	Variants	Predicted effect	Reference
IL-10	rs1800896 −819 T > C	*Susceptibility* The frequency of TT genotype was significantly increased ($p < 0.05$) in PCOS group	[23]
		Clinical manifestations CT and TT genotypes were associated with lower total cholesterol and triglyceride levels in PCOS patients ($p < 0.05$)	[38]
	rs1800871 −1082 A > G	*Susceptibility* G allele was significantly increased among PCOS patients ($p < 0.01$), while A allele was significantly increased ($p < 0.001$) in controls	[23]
		Clinical manifestations GA and AA genotypes were associated with lower total cholesterol and triglyceride levels ($p < 0.05$)	[38]
	rs1800872 −592 C > A	*Susceptibility* AA genotype carriers had increased risk of PCOS ($p = 0.001$)	[39]
		Clinical manifestations CA genotype was associated with lower total cholesterol and triglyceride levels ($p < 0.05$)	[38]
IL-1β	rs16944 −511 T > C	*Susceptibility* Both TT genotype frequency and T allele frequency were significantly higher in PCOS patients than controls (both p < 0.01)	[40]
		Susceptibility CC genotype frequency was significantly higher in PCOS patients than controls ($p < 0.001$)	[24]
		Clinical manifestations T allele showed significant association with several metabolic features associated with PCOS ($p < 0.05$ for all analyses)	[41]
		Clinical manifestations Both TT genotype frequency and T allele frequency were significantly higher in obese PCOS patients than nonobese patients ($p < 0.05$ for all analyses)	[42]
IL-18	rs187238 −137 C > G	*Clinical manifestations* C allele frequencies were significantly higher in PCOS patients with IR than PCOS patients without IR ($p = 0.048$)	[43]
		Susceptibility CC and GC genotypes were associated with increased risk of developing PCOS ($p < 0.05$)	[44]
		Clinical manifestations PCOS patients with GG genotype had a significantly increased risk of impaired glucose regulation compared to C allele carriers ($p < 0.05$)	[45]
IL-1α	rs1800587 −889 C > T	*Susceptibility* The distribution of genotype frequencies was statistically different in women with PCOS compared to controls ($p = 0.04$) *Clinical manifestations* The serum level of FSH and subsequent LH/FSH ratio correlated with the polymorphism within the PCOS group ($p = 0.005$ and 0.01, respectively)	[46]

Table 1.
The associations between genetic polymorphisms in genes related to inflammatory markers and PCOS risk or clinical manifestations.

3. Oxidative stress in PCOS

OS has been a highly researched topic in the last two decades, due to the discovery that imbalance between oxidants and antioxidants results in an abnormal redox state of cells. This state is involved in the development of many diseases, such as diabetes, cancer, atherosclerosis, depression, PCOS, and a few neurological diseases. OS reflects an imbalance between production and scavenging of reactive oxygen (ROS) and nitrogen species (RNS). The ROS include superoxide radical, hydrogen peroxide, and hydroxyl radical, and the RNS include NO and its metabolites. Some ROS can also act as cellular messengers. The peroxides and free radicals are unstable and highly reactive and can damage different cell components. The most worrying long-term effects are caused by the damage to the DNA [47, 48].

OS is considered as a potential inducing factor in the PCOS pathogenesis. In most studies, PCOS patients present with higher levels of OS than controls. However, results often vary, mainly due to the employment of different markers and evaluation of the same marker in different sources and even with different investigation methods. Moreover, OS is not necessarily associated only with PCOS pathogenesis, since many clinical manifestations of PCOS, like hyperandrogenism, obesity, and IR, may be a contributing factor in the development of the local and systemic OS, which may then reciprocally worsen those metabolic abnormalities [49].

Levels of molecular markers that could reflect the systemic OS, such as oxidized low-density lipoprotein, malondialdehyde, thiobarbituric reactive substances, and advanced oxidation protein products, were significantly increased in obese people as compared with controls. On the other hand, markers that could reflect antioxidant activity such as glutathione peroxidase (GPx) and superoxide dismutase (SOD) were significantly decreased in obese as compared to controls. However, obesity is probably only a contributing factor to OS in PCOS. When obese patients are ruled out based on BMI, nonobese women with PCOS still have higher OS markers than healthy controls [47].

One other important contributing factor to OS in PCOS women is IR. The mechanism behind this is that hyperglycemia and higher levels of free fatty acids lead to ROS production. On the other hand, OS can be an important factor in the development of IR. There is a well-known phenomenon called OS-induced IR. The full mechanism behind it is still unknown, but it was reported in multiple studies that exposure to OS inhibits insulin-stimulated glucose uptake, glycogen, and protein synthesis. Increased OS activates various protein kinases, which induce serine or threonine phosphorylation on insulin receptor substrate (IRS) instead of normal tyrosine phosphorylation. This reduces the ability of the IRS to combine with the insulin receptor and suppresses its activation of downstream phosphatidylinositol 3-kinase. Furthermore, the wrong phosphorylation could also induce the degradation of IRS. Insulin signaling pathways could also be activated by OS through Jun N-terminal kinase/stress-activated protein kinase signaling pathway and inflammatory signaling pathway (IκB kinase/NF-κB), leading to IR via post-insulin receptor defect [47].

Antioxidants, on the other hand, are a class of molecules that can reduce the destructive effects of free radicals. In general, we can divide antioxidants into two groups: enzymatic like (SOD, catalase (CAT), GPx, glutathione reductase, paraoxonase 1 (PON-1)) and nonenzymatic (glutathione, alfa-tocopherol, ascorbate, and beta-carotene). These antioxidants have already been reported to have an important role in the female reproductive system and the pathogenesis of female infertility [50].

In general, chemical substances used for evaluation of OS status can be divided into chemical components modified by ROS, ROS scavenging enzymes or antioxidative chemicals, and transcription factors regulating ROS production. Many studies tried to evaluate OS markers in PCOS women, but due to small study groups, results often varied. A meta-analysis of these markers was published in 2013. It encompassed 63 different studies and included 4933 PCOS patients and 3671 controls. It showed that the serum concentrations of several promoters and by-products of OS were significantly increased in patients with PCOS compared with control women. Homocysteine concentrations were 23% higher in PCOS patients than control women according to this meta-analysis. Homocysteine induces OS by promoting ROS production, and its high serum level makes a person more prone to endothelial cell injury. A 47% increase was noticed in malondialdehyde, an end-product of lipid peroxidation and a useful and frequently used marker of OS. On the other hand, some circulating antioxidant markers were decreased in PCOS. Glutathione, which plays a key protective role against OS, was decreased by 50%. A similar decrease was noticed in the activity of PON-1, which is an antioxidant enzyme that prevents the oxidation of lipoproteins and hydrolyzes atherogenic products of oxidative lipid modification such as phospholipid peroxides and cholesterol ester hydroperoxides. Contrary to what was expected, a meta-analysis found an increase in the SOD activity in PCOS patients. An increase in that potent protective enzyme, scavenging superoxide anion radical, may be interpreted as a compensatory mechanism in response to the increased production of other oxidant molecules. This meta-analysis did not find significant differences among patients with PCOS and control women in NO levels, GPx activity, and total antioxidant capacity, although many individual studies reported significant differences [49]. A similar increase in some antioxidative enzymes has already been described in few other studies. A study published in 2018 noticed a significant increase in CAT and SOD activity, and their interpretation of those results focused on an inner stress-counterbalanced effect [51].

Since a large proportion of studies indicated an important imbalance in the oxidative status of patients with PCOS, there have been a few attempts to treat patients with antioxidants. A single-blind randomized control trial involving 200 patients with PCOS was published in 2018. Patients were randomized into intervention and control groups, and baseline serum levels of OS markers, antioxidant enzymes, vitamins, and minerals were determined. Antioxidant supplementation and placebo were given to the intervention and control groups, respectively. All patients had ovulation induction with clomiphene and were followed up for 6 months. There was statistically significant difference in the serum levels of OS marker, antioxidant enzymes, vitamins, and minerals between the two groups. Not only did the antioxidant supplementation significantly improve oxidative status in those patients, but it also significantly affected pregnancy rate [52]. A recent study has also shown promising results with the mitochondria-targeted antioxidant for PCOS IR in animal model [53].

Researches have already confirmed that genetic changes in key antioxidant enzymes and inflammatory mediators can affect the individual's defense ability against OS and their predisposition to inflammation. In **Table 2**, we summarized the main studies which pointed out positive associations between different polymorphisms in genes related to previously described oxidative markers and antioxidant enzymes and PCOS risk or clinical manifestations. At the time of the writing, we could not find any study that explored the relationship between polymorphisms in those genes and treatment response.

Gene	Variants	Predicted effect	Reference
PON-1	rs705379 −108 C > T	*Susceptibility* Genotype distribution differed significantly between PCOS patients and controls ($p < 0.05$)	[54]
		Susceptibility Association with increased risk of PCOS was observed in three genetic models: allelic comparison, homozygote comparison, and recessive comparison ($p < 0.05$ for all analyses)	[55]
		Susceptibility Results show a significant association between PCOS and this polymorphism (for T vs. C: $p = 0.012$, for TT vs. CC: $p = 0.005$, for TT vs. TC+CC: $p = 0.01$)	[56]
		Susceptibility The TT genotype was more frequent in PCOS patients than in controls ($p < 0.01$) *Clinical manifestations* Free androgen index levels were higher in patients with TT genotype ($p < 0.05$)	[57]
	rs854560 163 T > A	*Susceptibility* Genotype and allele frequency distributions differed significantly between lean controls and lean PCOS women ($p < 0.05$). This polymorphism reduced the risk of PCOS in lean but not in obese Indian women ($p < 0.05$) *Clinical manifestations* This polymorphism influenced glucose metabolism, lipid parameters, and hyperandrogenemia in the study group ($p < 0.05$ for all analyses)	[58]
		Susceptibility The association between polymorphism and a decreased risk of PCOS was found in dominant model ($p < 0.05$)	[55]
	rs662 575 A > G	*Susceptibility* GG genotype and G allele frequencies were higher in patients with PCOS than in control women ($p < 0.05$) *Clinical manifestations* Compared with patients with AA genotype, patients with GG or AG genotype had significantly higher waist circumference and fasting insulin and triglyceride levels, patients with GG genotype had significantly higher waist-to-hip ratio, and patients with AG genotype had significantly higher HOMA index ($p < 0.05$ for all analyses)	[59]
		Susceptibility Women with AG or GG genotypes had a 2.5-fold increased risk of PCOS compared to AA genotype ($p = 0.03$)	[60]
		Susceptibility Polymorphism was significantly associated with PCOS (for G allele vs. A allele: $p = 0.02$, for GG+AG vs. AA: $p = 0.043$)	[56]
		Susceptibility GG genotype and G allele frequencies were higher in PCOS than in controls ($p < 0.05$ for all analyses) *Clinical manifestations* Testosterone, free androgen index, and dehydroepiandrosterone sulfate levels were higher in patients with GG than in patients with the wild or the heterozygous genotype group ($p < 0.05$ for all analyses)	[57]

Gene	Variants	Predicted effect	Reference
GSTM1	deletion	*Clinical manifestations* Adolescent girls with PCOS with GSTM1-null genotype (no active alleles present) presented significantly lower testosterone concentrations than those with the GSTM1-active genotype ($p < 0.05$)	[61]
SOD2	rs4880 47 T > C	*Susceptibility* The prevalence of the C allele was significantly greater in PCOS patients than in controls ($p < 0.05$) *Clinical manifestations* Patients carrying the C allele had significantly higher serum LH levels and ratio of LH to FSH than patients with the TT genotype ($p < 0.05$ for all analyses)	[62]

Table 2.
Associations between genetic polymorphisms in antioxidant genes and PCOS risk or clinical manifestations.

4. Interplay between oxidative stress and chronic inflammation

OS and inflammation are closely related pathophysiological processes, one of which can be easily induced by another. They usually occur simultaneously, and because of that, it is hard to distinguish them completely in pathological conditions.

On the one hand, inflammatory processes can induce OS through different pathways. Phagocytic cells like neutrophils and macrophages produce large amounts of ROS and RNS to destroy invading agents. During pathological inflammatory conditions, there may be an exaggerated generation of these reactive species. Some of those diffuse out of their phagocytic cells and can induce localized OS. The similar process happens in nonphagocytic cells, which can also produce reactive species in response to proinflammatory cytokines [63]. Recent studies have also shown that activation of multiple Toll-like receptors produces unbalance between proinflammatory and anti-inflammatory cytokines, and this leads to the insurgence of OS [64]. Moreover, the proinflammatory cytokine IL-6 has been found to produce ROS through increased expression of nicotinamide adenine dinucleotide phosphate oxidase 4 (NOX4) in non-small cell lung cancer. Similarly, the NOX4 overexpression can then enhance IL-6 production, and that forms a positive reciprocal feedback loop between these two mediators of inflammation and OS [63].

On the other hand, OS has been shown to induce inflammation. Growth factors and chemokines produced by inflammatory cells induce the overexpression of several transcription factors, such as NF-κB, signal transducer and activator of transcription 3 (STAT3), activating protein-1 (AP-1), and hypoxia-inducible factor-1 (HIF-1). They also activate redox-sensitive signal transduction pathways such as c-Jun N-terminal kinase and p38 mitogen-activated protein kinase (MAPK) [65, 66]. OS also plays an important role in the activation of the NLRP3 inflammasome, which promotes the maturation and secretion of proinflammatory cytokines IL-1β, IL-18, and IFNγ and activates NF-κB. NLRP3 inflammasome can be activated in multiple ways by OS. Besides activation by transcription factors, NLRP3 can be activated by ROS released from the damaged mitochondria and oxidized mitochondrial DNA during apoptosis. In conditions of OS, the ROS causes the thioredoxin-interacting protein, an inhibitor of endogenous antioxidant thioredoxin, to dissociate from thioredoxin and to bind with NLRP3 leading to additional activation of NLRP3 inflammasome [63]. Another possible mechanism for NLRP3 inflammasome activation is through ROS-induced DNA base modifications. Moreover, the OS-induced oxidation of the extracellular redox potential of plasma cysteine and its disulfide cysteine has been shown to trigger monocyte adhesion to vascular endothelial cells, activate NF-κB, and increase the expression of proinflammatory cytokine IL-1β [63]. OS also induces heat shock proteins, which in turn stimulate the production of proinflammatory cytokines and expression of the adhesion molecules like E-selectin, intercellular adhesion molecule 1, and vascular cell adhesion molecule 1 [66].

All these pathways seem to connect OS and inflammation into a self-perpetuating cycle. In pathological conditions where OS is the primary abnormality, inflammation will eventually develop and will further accentuate OS. Conversely, when inflammation is the main abnormality, OS will develop and will increase the damage from inflammation. Therefore identification of the primary abnormality could be extremely important in many conditions because its treatment could resolve additional problems from secondary OS or inflammation [63].

When it comes to PCOS, there is not yet enough evidence to confirm that either OS or inflammation is the main abnormality. However, the majority of studies agree that both phenomena at least play an important role in the clinical manifestations of that syndrome. One clinical manifestation that has been studied for its role in both OS and inflammation is obesity. Adipocytes have been identified as a source of proinflammatory cytokines which can then stimulate the production of ROS and RNS by macrophages and monocytes. One possible trigger for adipose tissue production of those cytokines is hypoxia. Adipose tissue hypoxia may underlie the dysregulated production of adipocytokines. In obese patients, adipose tissue also has the secretory capacity of angiotensin II, which stimulates nicotinamide adenine dinucleotide phosphate (NADPH) oxidase activity. NADPH oxidase comprises the major route for ROS production in adipocytes. The second clinical manifestation that has already been connected with both OS and inflammation is IR. OS has been recently recognized as one of the key mechanisms in IR. The hypothesis that inflammation is causally linked to IR is supported by clinical evidence of correlations between inflammatory markers and measures of IR and also by biochemical evidence indicating that proinflammatory markers can interfere with insulin action by directly inhibiting insulin receptors [67]. IR then plays a key role in hyperandrogenemia, likely due to compensatory hyperinsulinemia. Insulin is reported to stimulate ovarian androgen secretion directly alone and/or through augment LH-stimulated androgen secretion. Studies show that excessive activation of androgen receptor may provoke systemic OS. In vitro, OS was also reported to enhance the activities of ovarian steroidogenesis enzymes [47, 68]. Considering all previously discussed pathways, it seems that all the described changes—inflammation, OS, obesity, IR, and hyperandrogenism—interact among themselves and amplify each other in PCOS patients [69].

5. Conclusions

The majority of studies confirm that PCOS patients have elevated levels of OS and inflammatory mediators and that OS and inflammation may play an important role in the pathogenesis of the syndrome and its clinical manifestations. There are also several possible pathways how those two processes could form positive reciprocal feedback between each other and also between clinical manifestations of PCOS, such as obesity, IR, and hyperandrogenism.

Given the importance of OS and inflammation in PCOS, many researchers have tried to find associations between different polymorphisms in genes related to these pathways and PCOS risk, clinical manifestations, or treatment response. Evidence shows that different genetic polymorphisms in those pathways have an important role in susceptibility for the development of PCOS and that they greatly influence its clinical manifestations. There is still a lack of studies that would evaluate how those polymorphisms affect individual treatment response. Large pharmacogenetic studies would improve our understanding of PCOS pathogenesis, and they could identify polymorphisms potentially used as a predictive biomarker for evaluating the risk for developing PCOS and for predicting treatment response in an individual patient.

Abbreviations

AP-1	activating protein-1
ASC	apoptosis-associated speck-like protein
BMI	body mass index
CAT	catalase
CRP	C-reactive protein
CVD	cardiovascular disease
FF	follicular fluid
FSH	follicle-stimulating hormoneGLP-1glucagon-like peptide 1
GPx	glutathione peroxidase
HIF-1	hypoxia-inducible factor-1
HOMA	homeostatic model assessment
IFNγ	interferon gamma
IL-1	interleukin 1
IL-6	interleukin 6
IL-8	interleukin 8
IL-10	interleukin 10
IL-12	interleukin 12
IL-18	interleukin 18
IR	insulin resistance
IRS	insulin receptor substrate
LH	luteinizing hormone
MAPK	mitogen-activated protein kinase
MS	metabolic syndrome
NF-κB	nuclear factor κBNOnitric oxide
NOX4	nicotinamide adenine dinucleotide phosphate oxidase 4
OS	oxidative stress
PCOS	polycystic ovary syndrome
PON-1	paraoxonase 1
RNS	reactive nitrogen species
ROS	reactive oxygen species
SHBG	sex hormone-binding globulin
SOD	superoxide dismutase
STAT3	signal transducer and activator of transcription 3
TNFα	tumor necrosis factor alpha

Author details

Rok Herman[1], Mojca Jensterle Sever[2,3], Andrej Janež[2,3] and Vita Dolžan[1]*

1 Pharmacogenetics Laboratory, Faculty of Medicine, Institute of Biochemistry, University of Ljubljana, Slovenia

2 Department of Endocrinology, Diabetes and Metabolic Diseases, University Medical Centre Ljubljana, Slovenia

3 Department of Internal Medicine, Faculty of Medicine, University of Ljubljana, Slovenia

*Address all correspondence to: vita.dolzan@mf.uni-lj.si

References

[1] Sheehan MT. Polycystic ovarian syndrome: Diagnosis and management. Clinical Medicine & Research. 2004;**2**(1):13-27

[2] Kabel AM. Polycystic ovarian syndrome: Insights into pathogenesis, diagnosis, prognosis, pharmacological and non-pharmacological treatment. Journal of Pharmacological Reports. 2016;**1**:103

[3] Williams T, Mortada R, Porter S. Diagnosis and treatment of polycystic ovary syndrome. American Family Physician. 2016;**94**(2):106-113

[4] Jensterle M, Kravos NA, Goričar K, Janez A. Short-term effectiveness of low dose liraglutide in combination with metformin versus high dose liraglutide alone in treatment of obese PCOS: Randomized trial. BMC Endocrine Disorders. 31 Jan 2017;**17**(1):5

[5] Brännström M. Potential role of cytokines in ovarian physiology: The case for Interleukin-1. The Ovary. 2004. pp. 261-271

[6] Duleba AJ, Dokras A. Is PCOS an inflammatory process? Fertility and Sterility. 2012;**97**(1):7-12

[7] Caserta D, Adducchio G, Picchia S, Ralli E, Matteucci E, Moscarini M. Metabolic syndrome and polycystic ovary syndrome: An intriguing overlapping. Gynecological Endocrinology. 2014;**30**(6):397-402

[8] Escobar-Morreale HF, Luque-Ramírez M, González F. Circulating inflammatory markers in polycystic ovary syndrome: A systematic review and meta-analysis. Fertility and Sterility. 1 Mar 2011;**95**(3):1048-1058.e1-2

[9] Ebejer K, Calleja-Agius J. The role of cytokines in polycystic ovarian syndrome. Gynecological Endocrinology. 2013;**29**(6):536-540

[10] Spritzer PM, Lecke SB, Satler F, Morsch DM. Adipose tissue dysfunction, adipokines, and low-grade chronic inflammation in polycystic ovary syndrome. Reproduction. 2015;**149**(5):R219-R227

[11] Kelly CCJ, Lyall H, Petrie JR, Gould GW, Connell JMC, Sattar N. Low grade chronic inflammation in women with polycystic ovarian syndrome. The Journal of Clinical Endocrinology and Metabolism. 2001;**86**(6):2453-2455

[12] Diamanti-Kandarakis E, Paterakis T, Alexandraki K, Piperi C, Aessopos A, Katsikis I, et al. Indices of low-grade chronic inflammation in polycystic ovary syndrome and the beneficial effect of metformin. Human Reproduction. 2006;**21**(6):1426-1431

[13] Morin-Papunen L, Rautio K, Ruokonen A, Hedberg P, Puukka M, Tapanainen JS. Metformin reduces serum C-reactive protein levels in women with polycystic ovary syndrome. The Journal of Clinical Endocrinology and Metabolism. 2003;**88**(10):4649-4654

[14] Sathyapalan T, Kilpatrick ES, Coady AM, Atkin SL. The effect of atorvastatin in patients with polycystic ovary syndrome: A randomized double-blind placebo-controlled study. The Journal of Clinical Endocrinology and Metabolism. 2009;**94**(1):103-108

[15] Webb MA, Mani H, Robertson SJ, Waller HL, Webb DR, Edwardson CL, et al. Moderate increases in daily step count are associated with reduced IL6 and CRP in women with PCOS. Endocrine Connections. 1 Dec 2018;7(12):1442-1447

[16] Artimani T, Karimi J, Mehdizadeh M, Yavangi M,

Khanlarzadeh E, Ghorbani M, et al. Evaluation of pro-oxidant-antioxidant balance (PAB) and its association with inflammatory cytokines in polycystic ovary syndrome (PCOS). Gynecological Endocrinology. 2018;**34**(2):148-152

[17] Gao L, Gu Y, Yin X. High serum tumor necrosis factor-alpha levels in women with polycystic ovary syndrome: A meta-analysis. PLoS One. 2016;**11**(10):e0164021

[18] Sathyapalan T, Atkin SL. Mediators of inflammation in polycystic ovary syndrome in relation to adiposity. Mediators of Inflammation. 2010;**2010**: 758656

[19] Dawood A, Alkafrawy N, Saleh S, Noreldin R, Zewain S. The relationship between IL-18 and atherosclerotic cardiovascular risk in Egyptian lean women with polycystic ovary syndrome. Gynecological Endocrinology. 2018;**34**(4):294-297

[20] Yang Y, Qiao J, Li R, Li MZ. Is interleukin-18 associated with polycystic ovary syndrome? Reproductive Biology and Endocrinology. 18 Jan 2011;**9**:7

[21] Peng Z, Sun Y, Lv X, Zhang H, Liu C, Dai S. Interleukin-6 levels in women with polycystic ovary syndrome: A systematic review and meta-analysis. PLoS One [Internet]. 2016;**11**(2):e0148531. Available from: https://www.ncbi.nlm.nih.gov/pubmed/26849353

[22] Fulghesu AM, Sanna F, Uda S, Magnini R, Portoghese E, Batetta B. Il-6 serum levels and production is related to an altered immune response in polycystic ovary syndrome girls with insulin resistance. Mediators of Inflammation. 2011;**2011**:389317

[23] Talaat RM, Mohamed YA, Mohamad EH, Elsharkawy M, Guirgis AA. Interleukin 10 (−1082 G/A) and (−819 C/T) gene polymorphisms in Egyptian women with polycystic ovary syndrome (PCOS). Meta Gene. 2016;**9**: 254-258

[24] Mu Y, Liu J, Wang B, Wen Q, Wang J, Yan J, et al. Interleukin 1 beta (IL-1β) promoter C [−511] T polymorphism but not C [+3953] T polymorphism is associated with polycystic ovary syndrome. Endocrine. 2010;**37**(1):71-75

[25] Yang Y, Wang H, Kouadir M, Song H, Shi F. Recent advances in the mechanisms of NLRP3 inflammasome activation and its inhibitors. Cell Death and Disease. 12 Feb 2019;**10**(2):128

[26] Wang F, Wang S, Zhang Z, Lin Q, Liu Y, Xiao Y, et al. Activation of NLRP3 inflammasome in the ovaries during the development and treatment of polycystic ovary syndrome. International Journal of Clinical and Experimental Pathology. 2017;**10**(5): 5022-5030

[27] Abate E, Blomgran R, Verma D, Lerm M, Fredrikson M, Belayneh M, et al. Polymorphisms in CARD8 and NLRP3 are associated with extrapulmonary TB and poor clinical outcome in active TB in Ethiopia. Scientific Reports. 28 Feb 2019;**9**(1): 3126

[28] Deepika MLN, Reddy KR, Yashwanth A, Rani VU, Latha KP, Jahan P. TNF-α haplotype association with polycystic ovary syndrome—A South Indian study. Journal of Assisted Reproduction and Genetics. 2013;**30** (11):1493-503

[29] Yun JH, Choi JW, Lee KJ, Shin JS, Baek KH. The promoter −1031(T/C) polymorphism in tumor necrosis factor-alpha associated with polycystic ovary syndrome. Reproductive Biology and Endocrinology. 4 Oct 2011;**9**:131

[30] Diao X, Han T, Zhang Y, Ma J, Shi Y, Chen ZJ. Family association study between tumour necrosis factor a gene

polymorphisms and polycystic ovary syndrome in Han Chinese. Reproductive Biomedicine Online. 2014;**29**(5):581-587

[31] Thathapudi S, Kodati V, Erukkambattu J, Katragadda A, Addepally U, Hasan Q. Tumor necrosis factor-alpha and polycystic ovarian syndrome: A clinical, biochemical, and molecular genetic study. Genetic Testing and Molecular Biomarkers. 2014;**18**(9):605-609

[32] Li S, Zhao L, Wan X-H. A missense variant rs4645843 in *TNF-α* gene is a risk factor of polycystic ovary syndrome in the Uygur population. The Tohoku Journal of Experimental Medicine. 2017; **243**(2):95-100

[33] Tumu VR, Govatati S, Guruvaiah P, Deenadayal M, Shivaji S, Bhanoori M. An interleukin-6 gene promoter polymorphism is associated with polycystic ovary syndrome in South Indian women. Journal of Assisted Reproduction and Genetics. 2013;**30** (12):1541-1546

[34] Chen L, Zhang Z, Huang J, Jin M. Association between rs1800795 polymorphism in the interleukin-6 gene and the risk of polycystic ovary syndrome: A meta-analysis. Medicine. 2018;**97**(29):e11558

[35] Villuendas G, San Millán JL, Sancho J, Escobar-Morreale HF. The −597 G→A and −174 G→C polymorphisms in the promoter of the IL-6 gene are associated with hyperandrogenism. The Journal of Clinical Endocrinology and Metabolism. 2002;**87**(3):1134-1141

[36] Erdogan M, Karadeniz M, Berdeli A, Alper G, Caglayan O, Yilmaz C. The relationship of the interleukin-6 −174 G > C gene polymorphism with oxidative stress markers in Turkish polycystic ovary syndrome patients. Journal of Endocrinological Investigation. 2008; **31**(7):624-629

[37] Eser B, Islimye Taskin M, Hismiogullari AA, Aksit H, Bodur AS. The effects of IL-1A and IL-6 genes polymorphisms on gene expressions, hormonal and biochemical parameters in polycystic ovary syndrome. Journal of Obstetrics and Gynaecology. 2017;**37**(3): 358-362

[38] Sóter MO, Ferreira CN, Sales MF, Candido AL, Reis FM, Milagres KS, et al. Peripheral blood-derived cytokine gene polymorphisms and metabolic profile in women with polycystic ovary syndrome. Cytokine. 2015;**76**(2):227-235

[39] Xing G, Sun Y, Wang F, Gao G, Zhou X. Role of interleukin-10 polymorphisms and haplotypes in polycystic ovary syndrome risk. International Journal of Clinical and Experimental Pathology. 2017;**10**(7): 7956-7961. Available from: http://www.ijcep.com/files/ijcep0054344.pdf

[40] Xia YH, Yao L, Zhang ZX. Correlation between IL-1β, IL-1Ra gene polymorphism and occurrence of polycystic ovary syndrome infertility. Asian Pacific Journal of Tropical Medicine. 2013;**6**(3):232-236

[41] Rashid N, Nigam A, Saxena P, Jain SK, Wajid S. Association of IL-1β, IL-1Ra and FABP1 gene polymorphisms with the metabolic features of polycystic ovary syndrome. Inflammation Research. 2017;**66**(7):621-636

[42] Yang Y, Qiao J, Li M. Correlation between interleukin-1 and the obesity of polycystic ovary syndrome. Zhonghua Fu Chan Ke Za Zhi. 2012;**47**(1):9-13

[43] Yang Y, Qiao J, Li MZ. Association of polymorphisms of interleukin-18 gene promoter region with polycystic ovary syndrome in Chinese population. Reproductive Biology and Endocrinology. 22 Oct 2010;**8**:125

[44] Wang Q, Tan Z, Zhang H, Min R, Cheng Z, Wei L. Association of IL-18 polymorphisms with risk of polycystic

ovary syndrome in a han population of China. Biomedical Research. 2018;**29**: 108-112

[45] Kim JW, Lee MH, Park JE, Yoon TK, Lee WS, Shim SH. Association of IL-18 genotype with impaired glucose regulation in Korean women with polycystic ovary syndrome. European Journal of Obstetrics, Gynecology, and Reproductive Biology. 2012;**161**(1):51-55

[46] Kolbus A, Walch K, Nagele F, Wenzl R, Unfried G, Huber JC. Interleukin-1 alpha but not interleukin-1 beta gene polymorphism is associated with polycystic ovary syndrome. Journal of Reproductive Immunology. 2007;**73** (2):188-193

[47] Zuo T, Zhu M, Xu W. Roles of oxidative stress in polycystic ovary syndrome and cancers. Oxidative Medicine and Cellular Longevity. 2016; **2016**:8589318

[48] Desai V, Prasad NR, Manohar SM, Sachan A, Lakshmi Narasimha SRPV, Bitla ARR. Oxidative stress in non-obese women with polycystic ovarian syndrome. Journal of Clinical and Diagnostic Research. 2014;**8**(7):CC01-3

[49] Murri M, Luque-ramírez M, Insenser M, Ojeda-ojeda M, Escobar-morreale HF. Circulating markers of oxidative stress and polycystic ovary syndrome (pcos): A systematic review and meta-analysis. Human Reproduction Update. 2013;**19**(3): 268-288

[50] Sulaiman MA, Al-Farsi YM, Al-Khaduri MM, Saleh J, Waly MI. Polycystic ovarian syndrome is linked to increased oxidative stress in Omani women. International Journal of Women's Health. 2018;**10**:763-771. Available from: https://www.ncbi.nlm.nih.gov/pubmed/30568513

[51] Gyftaki R, Gougoura S, Kalogeris N, Loi V, Koukoulis G, Vryonidou A. Oxidative stress markers in women with polycystic ovary syndrome without insulin resistance. Endocrine Abstracts. 2018;**56**:P950. Available from: https://www.endocrine-abstracts.org/ea/0056/ea0056p950.htm

[52] Panti AA, Shehu CE, Saidu Y, Tunau KA, Nwobodo EI, Jimoh A, et al. Oxidative stress and outcome of antioxidant supplementation in patients with polycystic ovarian syndrome (PCOS). International Journal of Reproduction, Contraception, Obstetrics and Gynecology. 2016;**48**(3):185-190

[53] Ding Y, Jiang Z, Xia B, Zhang L, Zhang C, Leng J. Mitochondria-targeted antioxidant therapy for an animal model of PCOS-IR. International Journal of Molecular Medicine. 2019;**43**(1):316-324

[54] Knebel B, Janssen OE, Hahn S, Nitzgen U, Jacob S, Haas J, et al. Combined analyses of paraoxonase-1 and IGF-2 polymorphism in polycystic ovary syndrome. Deutsche Medizinische Wochenschrift. 2009;**134** (20):1040-1046

[55] Chen B, Wang Y, Lin W, Jiang H, Liu C, Dong C, et al. Association between Paraoxonase-1 (PON-1) polymorphisms and polycystic ovary syndrome susceptibility: A meta-analysis. International Journal of Clinical and Experimental Medicine. 2016;**9**(2):1490-1499

[56] Liu L, Yang J, Liu Q, Yan W, Wen Y. Risk association of polycystic ovary syndrome with paraoxonase 1 and TNF-α gene polymorphisms: A meta-analysis. International Journal of Clinical and Experimental Medicine. 2016;**9**(4): 7088-7101. Available from: http://www.ijcem.com/files/ijcem0018469.pdf

[57] Paltoglou G, Tavernarakis G, Christopoulos P, Vlassi M, Gazouli M, Deligeoroglou E, et al. PON1-108 TT and PON1-192 RR genotypes are more frequently encountered in Greek PCOS

than non-PCOS women, and are associated with hyperandrogenaemia. Clinical Endocrinology. 2013;**79**(2): 259-266

[58] Dadachanji R, Shaikh N, Khavale S, Patil A, Shah N, Mukherjee S. PON1 polymorphisms are associated with polycystic ovary syndrome susceptibility, related traits, and PON1 activity in Indian women with the syndrome. Fertility and Sterility. 2015; **104**(1):207-216

[59] Wang Y, Liu H, Fan P, Bai H, Zhang J, Zhang F. Evidence for association between paraoxonase 1 gene polymorphisms and polycystic ovarian syndrome in south-west Chinese women. European Journal of Endocrinology. 2012;**166**(5):877-885

[60] Nalkiran HS, Sahin SB, Ayaz T, Nalkiran I, Guzel AI, Eldes T, et al. Association of paraoxonase-1 L55M and Q192R polymorphisms with PCOS risk and potential risk factors for atherosclerosis. Biomarkers in Medicine. 2019;**13**(4):279-289

[61] Savic-Radojevic A, Mazibrada I, Djukic T, Stankovic ZB, Pljesa-Ercegovac M, Sedlecky K, et al. Glutathione S-transferase (GST) polymorphism could be an early marker in the development of polycystic ovary syndrome (PCOS)—An insight from non-obese and non-insulin resistant adolescents. Endokrynologia Polska. 2018;**69**(4):366-374

[62] Liu Q, Liu H, Bai H, Huang W, Zhang R, Tan J, et al. Association of SOD2 A16V and PON2 S311C polymorphisms with polycystic ovary syndrome in Chinese women. Journal of Endocrinological Investigation. 2019;**42**(8):909-921

[63] Biswas SK. Does the interdependence between oxidative stress and inflammation explain the antioxidant paradox? Oxidative Medicine and Cellular Longevity. 2016; **2016**:5698931

[64] Lavieri R, Piccioli P, Carta S, Delfino L, Castellani P, Rubartelli A. TLR costimulation causes oxidative stress with unbalance of proinflammatory and anti-inflammatory cytokine production. Journal of Immunology. 1 Jun 2014;**192**(11):5373-5381

[65] Hussain SP, Harris CC. Inflammation and cancer: An ancient link with novel potentials. International Journal of Cancer. 1 Dec 2007;**121**(11): 2373-2380

[66] Vaziri ND, Rodríguez-Iturbe B. Mechanisms of disease: Oxidative stress and inflammation in the pathogenesis of hypertension. Nature Clinical Practice Nephrology. 2006;**2**(10):582-593

[67] Adabimohazab R, Garfinkel A, Milam EC, Frosch O, Mangone A, Convit A. Does inflammation mediate the association between obesity and insulin resistance? Inflammation. 2016; **39**(3):994-1003

[68] Liu S, Navarro G, Mauvais-Jarvis F. Androgen excess produces systemic oxidative stress and predisposes to β-cell failure in female mice. PLoS One. 24 Jun 2010;**5**(6):e11302

[69] Fernández-Sánchez A, Madrigal-Santillán E, Bautista M, Esquivel-Soto J, Morales-González Á, Esquivel-Chirino C, et al. Inflammation, oxidative stress, and obesity. International Journal of Molecular Sciences. 2011;**12**(5): 3117-3132

Chapter 9

Computational Systems Analysis on Polycystic Ovarian Syndrome (PCOS)

Nor Afiqah-Aleng and Zeti-Azura Mohamed-Hussein

Abstract

Complex diseases are caused by a combination of genetic and environmental factors. Unraveling the molecular pathways from the genetic factors that affect a phenotype is always difficult, but in the case of complex diseases, this is further complicated since genetic factors in affected individuals might be different. Polycystic ovarian syndrome (PCOS) is an example of a complex disease with limited molecular information. Recently, PCOS molecular omics data have increasingly appeared in many publications. We conduct extensive bioinformatics analyses on the data and perform strong integration of experimental and computational biology to understand its complex biological systems in examining multiple interacting genes and their products. PCOS involves networks of genes, and to understand them, those networks must be mapped. This approach has emerged as powerful tools for studying complex diseases and been coined as network biology. Network biology encompasses wide range of network types including those based on physical interactions between and among cellular components and those baised on similarity among patients or diseases. Each of these offers distinct biological clues that may help scientists transform their cellular parts list into insights about complex diseases. This chapter will discuss some computational analysis aspects on the omics studies that have been conducted in PCOS.

Keywords: polycystic ovarian syndrome, PCOS, systems biology, computational systems biology, protein-protein interaction analysis, network biology, pathway analysis

1. Introduction

Findings have shown that most pathological conditions and diseases involve genetic components, in diseases such as cystic fibrosis, hemophilia, and sickle cell disease, are caused by mutations in a single gene [1–3]. However, there are many other common medical problems such as cardiovascular diseases, diabetes mellitus, obesity, and polycystic ovarian syndrome (PCOS), which are not caused by single mutations [4–7]. The etiologies of those problems are much more complex where these disorders are highly associated with multiple genes/proteins in combination with multifactor including genetics, environment, and lifestyle. Many efforts have been done to overcome the complexity of these medical problems.

Studying diseases at the molecular level is one of the efforts in understanding complex diseases. The emergence of biological technology has yielded great advances in deciphering the pathobiology of diseases by generating numerous large omics (genomics, transcriptomics, proteomics, and metabolomics) datasets. These data capture a wide range of disease phenomena including mutations, gene expression, protein expression, metabolite profiling, and genetic and physical interactions between biological molecules, where each dataset offers distinctive of knowledge to understand the diseases. Complex diseases are insufficient by a single level independent omics dataset since those diseases are regulated at multiple systems levels. They can be manifested by integrated omics analysis (integration of multi-omics data).

The multi-omics analysis has brought a new challenge to develop methods or pipelines, statistics, algorithms, and tools for integration, and the assistant of computational systems analysis is in great need. Implementing integrative analysis on these multiple omics data is the best way in deriving systematical and comprehensive views of diseases, achieving a better understanding of disease mechanisms and finding operable personalized health treatments. With the help of computational systems analysis, research in the field of biology and biomedicine has gained tremendous benefits over the past few decades.

Computational systems analysis connects interdisciplinary perspectives with mathematical, algorithms, statistical, modeling and simulations, data repository, and/or network visualizations using computational technique to investigate certain biological phenomenon or condition in a systems view. Currently, there are many studies on the integrated omics data and used network biology, which is one of the main techniques in computational systems analysis to obtain an overview at the systems level in elucidating the pathobiology of human diseases. Network biology could systematically connect all the molecules generated from the omics studies that have been identified to be related to the disease. Other than network biology, there are studies that used simulations approach to have a better understanding of diseases. Database development is another computational systems analysis that serves to provide overall information about the diseases. This chapter encompasses the computational systems analysis, such as network biology, simulations, and data repository, which have been used to understand the pathobiology of human diseases, particularly in PCOS.

2. Network biology in disease

Early biological experiments revealed that proteins, as the main agents of biological function, determine the phenotype of all organisms. In the advent of molecular biology, it is assumed that proteins do not naturally function in isolated forms; instead, they have interactions with one another and also with other molecules (e.g., DNA, RNA, and metabolites) that mediate metabolic, signaling and regulatory pathways, cellular processes, and organismal systems [8]. Most of the biological characteristics or phenotypes arise from the complex interactions between the cell's numerous constituents [9]. Any interruptions to the interactions between those molecules can disturb the normal behavior of the cells and contribute to the medical problems or diseases [10]. Thus, studies on network biology in disease are essential as it can be used to detect interrupter biological events since the network biology plays a role to perceive the biological role within the cells [11].

In network biology, there are two types of analysis that often be performed to understand the pathobiology of diseases, that is, protein-protein interaction and pathway analysis.

2.1 Protein-protein interaction analysis

Protein is a biological molecule that plays an important role in the molecular process in a cell. It acts as an enzyme for metabolic reaction, DNA replication, molecular transporter, antigen defensive system, and cell to cell information transmission [12]. Proteins physically interact with each other to perform a biological function in a cell. Protein-protein interaction (PPI) has become a valuable approach to study the molecular mechanisms of disease [13]. For example, non-metastatic and metastatic breast tumors, as well as the markers of metastasis, have been classified and identified by a network-based method. Based on this study, the said method is more effective because it enables detection of the genes that play a role in metastasis, which is not otherwise picked up during differential expression analysis [14]. Protein networks for type-1 diabetes were constructed by integrating GWAS data with the information from protein-protein interaction databases. Eight new genes were subsequently identified, hence providing better knowledge of the mechanism of type-1 diabetes [15]. Besides, new pathways have been defined from the protein network-based Huntington, giving a deeper understanding of the pathogenesis of Huntington disease [16]. These studies indicate that a network, particularly that of proteins, could be one of the powerful tools in understanding the molecular basis of diseases. Thus, this method could be applied to unveil the molecular basis of PCOS.

There are several approaches including yeast-2-hybrid (Y2H) and mass spectrometry (MS) that have been used to identify the PPI [17–20]. All approaches have generated large interactome and progressively identified PPI network in several organisms such as virus (herpes virus) [21], prokaryote (*Escherichia coli*) [22], eukaryote (yeast) [18–20], nematode [23], fruit fly [24], and human [25, 26]. These PPI datasets have been compiled and stored in PPI databases such as Biological General Repository for Interaction Datasets (BIOGRID) [27], Database of Interacting Proteins (DIP) [28], GeneMANIA [29], Human Integrated Protein-Protein Interaction Reference (HIPPIE) [30], Human Integrated Protein-Protein Human Protein Reference (HPRD) [31], Interologous Interaction Database (I2D) [32], IntAct [33], MIPS Mammalian Protein-Protein Interaction Database (MIPS) [34], Molecular Interaction database (MINT) [35], and STRING [36] (**Table 1**).

Combination of PPI forms a network consists of two main components, i.e. (1) node that represents protein and (2) edge that refers to interaction (**Figure 1**). PPI network has been applied for evolutionary study [45], gene/protein functional prediction [46], and also pathobiology of diseases [47, 48]. There are few analyses that can be applied using the PPI network approach, and PPI network topological analysis is one of the analyses that often are used to study the pathobiology of human diseases. Degree distribution, which is a fraction of a number of the interaction of a node with the number of the interactions in a network, is one of the components in the network topology that have been measured. A node that has a high degree distribution is known as a hub protein. A hub protein is hypothesized to code an essential gene that plays an important role in a cell. Any physical or chemical alterations that occur to this hub protein can interrupt the interaction with other proteins, disturb the normal behavior of the cells and associated to a disease. Previous study by Wachi et al. found that proteins encode for the upregulated genes in the lung squamous cell carcinoma tend to have higher degree distribution [49]. Jonsson and Bates also found

Database	Description	URL	Reference
Agile Protein Interactomes DataServer (APID)	Is a collection of integrated known validated protein interactomes from 400 species, including humans	http://apid.dep.usal.es/	[37]
BioGRID	Curates sets of genetic, physical, and chemical interactions in humans and all major organisms	https://thebiogrid.org/	[27]
Database of Interacting Protein (DIP)	Is manually curated by expert curators. This database stores experimental PPI data	https://dip.doe-mbi.ucla.edu	[38]
GeneMANIA	Contains known PPI interactions, which are derived from curated PPI databases and experiments. Predicts PPI interactions in six species, including humans	https://genemania.org/	[29]
Human Integrated Protein-Protein Interaction rEference (HIPPIE)	Contains only human PPI interactions from experiments and curated PPI databases	http://cbdm-01.zdv.uni-mainz.de/~mschaefer/hippie/	[30]
Information Hyperlinked over Proteins (iHOP)	Provides PPIs curated from literature mining	https://bio.tools/ihop	[39]
Human Protein Reference Database (HPRD)	Stores information regarding proteins in humans, including PPIs	https://www.hprd.org/	[31]
Interologous Interaction Database (I2D)	Contains integrated known, experimental, and predicted PPIs for humans and five other species	http://ophid.utoronto.ca/ophidv2.204/	[32]
InnateDB	Stores experimentally verified interactions between genes, proteins, and signaling pathways involved in the innate immune response to microbial infection in humans, mice, and bovines	https://www.innatedb.com/	[40]
IntAct Molecular Interaction Database (IntAct)	All interactions are retrieved from literature and eleven other PPI databases. Is curated by EMBL-EBI and other PPI database teams	https://www.ebi.ac.uk/intact/	[33]
Molecular INTeraction database (MINT)	Compiles experimentally verified PPIs curated from the scientific literature	https://mint.bio.uniroma2.it/	[41]
STRING	Is a PPI database that provides interaction evidence from known interactions (curated databases and experiments), predicted interactions (neighborhood, gene fusion, and co-occurrence), and others (coexpression and text-mining)	https://string-db.org/	[36]
The Extracellular Matrix Interaction Database (MatrixDB)	Stores interactions of extracellular matrix proteins, proteoglycans, and polysaccharides	http://matrixdb.univ-lyon1.fr/	[42]
The Human Protein Interaction Database (HPID)	Compiles proteins from BIND (this PPI database is not open access), DIP, and HPRD and predicts potential PPIs	http://wilab.inha.ac.kr/hpid/	[43]

Database	Description	URL	Reference
The International Molecular Exchange Consortium (IMEx)	Provides nonredundant PPI datasets from major PPI databases like BIND, IntAct, MINT, DIP, and MIPS	https://www.imexconsortium.org/	[44]
The Mammalian Protein-Protein Interaction Database (MIPS)	Compiles high-quality PPIs from experiments	http://mips.helmholtz-muenchen.de/proj/ppi/	[34]

Table 1.
List of PPI databases concerning humans.

346 proteins-related to cancer have two times higher degree connectivity compared to the non-cancer proteins [50]. Number of interaction among proteins that are related to disease in the Online Mendelian Inheritance in Man (OMIM) Morbid Map is higher than the interaction of non-disease proteins [51].

Linkage method is another network analysis that can be used to understand the pathobiology of human diseases [50, 52]. The basic hypothesis in this method is the two proteins (pairwise linkage) that interact with each other tend to be related to the same diseases. Enrichment analysis done by Oti et al. [53] has demonstrated that the proteins that interact with each other are significantly associated with the same diseases. By a pairwise linkage method, they also predicted that Janus kinase 3 (JAK3) as a protein that might be associated with severe combined immunodeficiency syndrome (SCID) as JAK3 directly interacts with proteins of lymphocyte specific protein-tyrosine (LCK), protein-tyrosine phosphatase (PTPRC), and interleukin 2 receptor (IL2RG) [53].

Clustering is also a technique in network analysis in human diseases. A cluster refers to a small group that has similar topological network properties [48, 54]. In this method, it is hypothesized that the proteins in a module tend to be associated with the same diseases. Clusters are identified using algorithms, and there are several clustering algorithms that have been developed to generate the clusters such as CFinder [55], clustering with overlapping neighborhood expansion (ClusterONE) [56], clustering based on maximal cliques (CMC) [57], clique percolation method (CPM) [58],

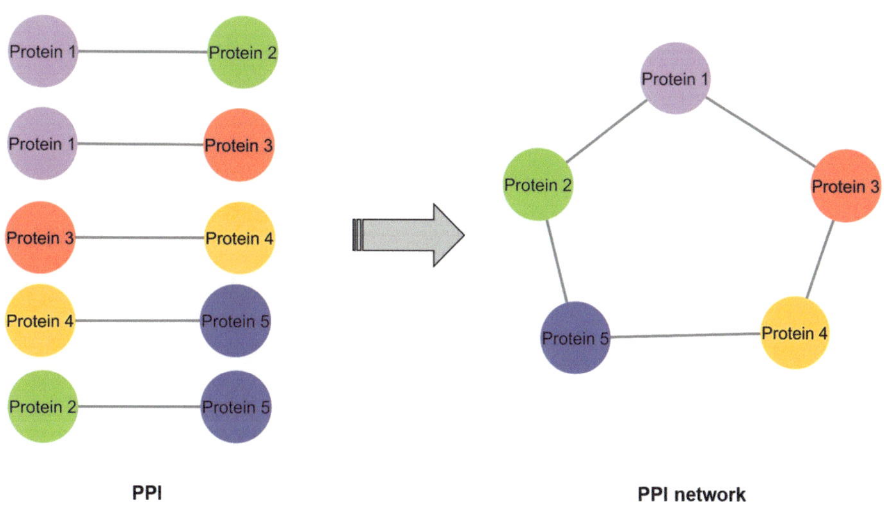

Figure 1.
PPI and PPI network. PPI network is formed from several PPI. The color of the nodes refers to the protein.

density-periphery based clustering (DPClus) [59], density-periphery overlapping-based clustering (DPClusO) [60, 61], identifying protein complex algorithm (IPCA) [62], local clique merging algorithm (LCMA) [63], restricted neighborhood search clustering (RNSC) [64], Markov clustering (MCL) [65], molecular complex detection (MCODE) [66], and so on. Wu et al. developed the clustering algorithm to identify the clusters, and they found that the proteins in the same clusters are associated with the same diseases [67]. Rezaei-Tavirani et al. identified clusters using ClusterONE algorithm to search for potential biomarkers in esophagus adenocarcinoma [68]. Xiao et al. also used clustering methods to identify the candidate proteins for endometriosis biomarkers by their own clustering algorithm and they found the majority of predicted biomarkers in the generated clusters involved in endometriosis pathway [69].

PPI network can be also applied to understand the association between diseases as clinically and there is the occurrence of comorbidity, which is a condition of a patient that is simultaneously affected more than one disease. Disease association network based on PPI analysis can be used as a framework to classify the disease, identify the risk of having other diseases, predict the effect of disease, and search for a more effective therapeutic technique for disease [70, 71]. There are few hypotheses in constructing the disease association network, and one of them is diseases can be associated when those diseases shared the proteins and interactions (**Figure 2**).

The components in a disease association network are similar to the PPI network. It consists of node and edge, where node refers to disease and edge is the interaction of disease. The first human disease network has been constructed among 867 diseases using PPI information by Goh et al. (**Figure 3**) [73]. This network has been used to understand how diseases comorbid to each other by identifying the shared proteins and interactions between the diseases [72]. The disease association network is also useful to predict the disease biomarkers. Ahmed et al. have successfully identified 73 potential biomarkers for neurological diseases, that is, Alzheimer's disease, epilepsy, and dyslexia, by integrating the protein-disease association with the PPI information [74].

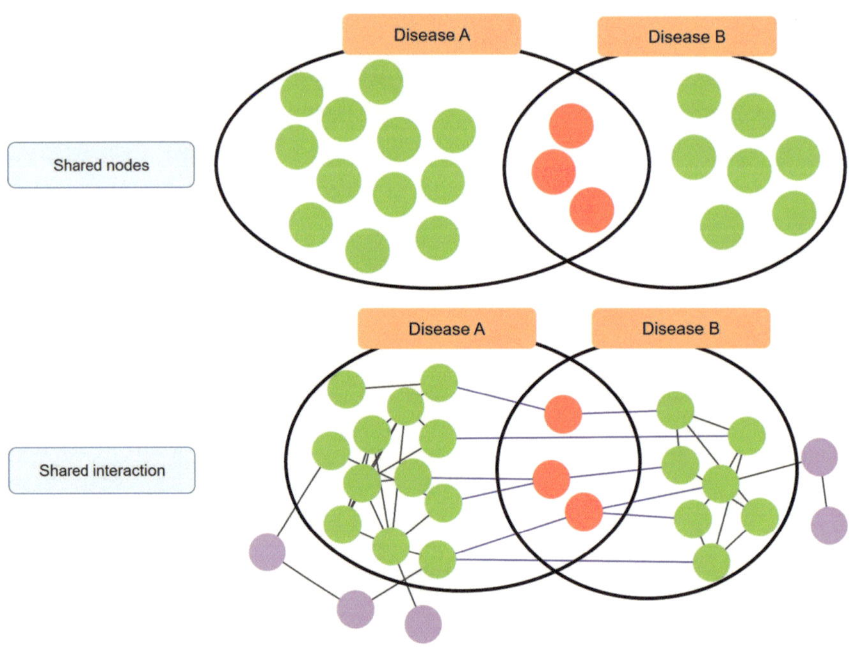

Figure 2.
Two different approaches to identify the association between diseases. The first approach used shared nodes (red nodes) between diseases. The second approach used shared interactions (blue edges) between disease-related proteins [72].

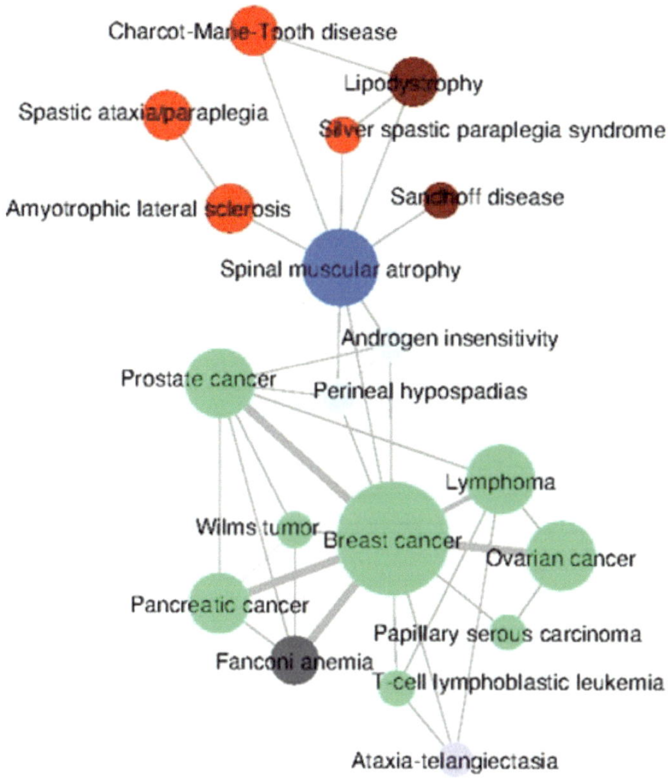

Figure 3.
Human disease association network. This network was constructed by Goh et al. using PPI information [73].

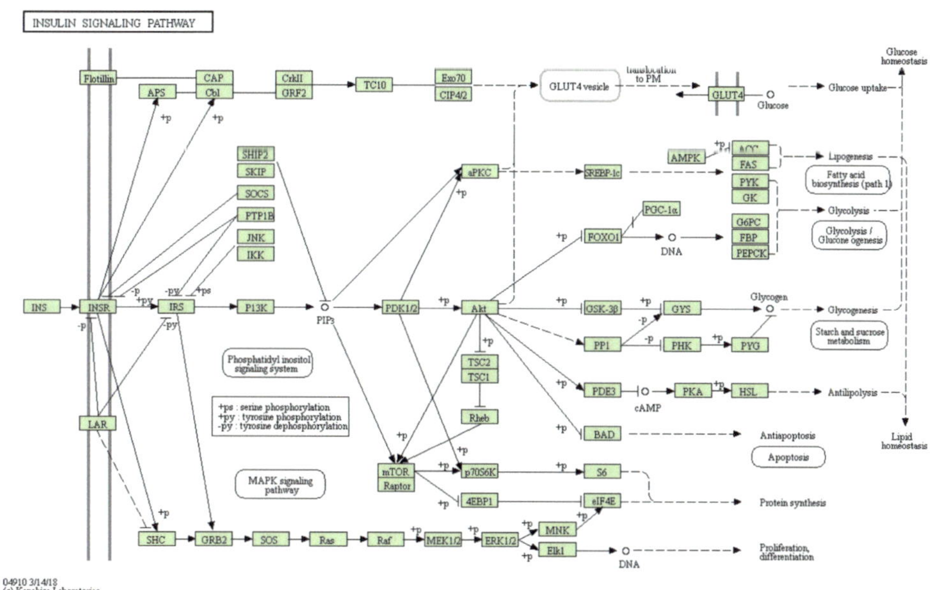

Figure 4.
Example of a biological pathway. This is the insulin signaling pathway that was retrieved from the KEGG database [80].

To summarize, PPI analysis is a powerful approach that can be applied to improve the understanding of the pathobiology of diseases, which in turn can appraise approaches to diagnose, prevent, and treat the diseases. The analysis of network properties can provide the opportunity to interpret the normal and altered biological behaviors that lead to diseases.

2.2 Pathway analysis

A pathway is a group of molecules that interact to perform the same biological function. PPI network has a type of node that is protein and the undirected network (**Figure 4**). Meanwhile, the pathway consists of a few types of nodes, which are signaling genes, proteins, complex, and metabolites, which are connected by several interactions such as activation, inhibition, binding, and others. A pathway depicts a mechanism in performing a specific biological activity in a cell. As a PPI network, a combination of several pathways forms a pathway network. Pathway information can be retrieved from several pathway databases such as Kyoto Encyclopedia of Genes and Genomes (KEGG) [75], Reactome [76], WikiPathways [77], BioCyc [78], and BioCarta [79]. **Table 2** shows databases that have pathway information in human.

There are three main types of pathways, that is, signaling, regulatory, and metabolic pathways. Signaling pathway visualizes the cellular response after receiving the extracellular signal. The signal transmission starts when the extracellular gives a signal to activate the receptor that is located in the cell surface. The activated receptor will bind to the signal and alter the intracellular molecules to respond [84]. Any disruption in the signaling pathway can cause disease since the cells cannot be normalized or properly respond when the signals are received [85]. Regulatory pathway displays the gene or protein expression in a cell, either it is upregulated or downregulated. The biological activities such as transcription, translation, and post-translational modification are among the activities that involve the regulatory pathway [86]. Meanwhile, in a metabolic pathway, the primer metabolite will be modified into another metabolite through a series of chemical reactions catalyzed by enzymes [87].

Pathway database such as KEGG also provides pathways that visualize the mechanisms of several complex diseases such as cancer, diabetes mellitus, Alzheimer's disease, Parkinson's disease, and so on [75]. Basically, a complex disease involves several pathways that include all signaling, regulatory, and metabolic pathways. The combination and the integration of several pathways with other types of data such as PPI is one of the valuable approaches that can be used to improve the understanding of complex disease mechanisms [88].

As an analogy, it is essential to have a diagram such as a circuit diagram for an electrician to understand the principle of electricity. A diagram such as a biological network is also important in the medical field to assist the researchers or clinicians to understand the mechanisms of diseases. The biological network can suggest a novel means of developing molecular therapies where the network is the target of therapy rather than individual molecules within the network.

3. Modeling and simulation

Mathematical modeling and computer simulation are another computational systems analysis that has been used to study disease progression and drug development [89, 90]. While the biological network is generally constructed in the static state using annotated genes, proteins, and metabolites and linked these molecules using information from PPI and pathway databases, modeling and simulation are constructed in quasi-steady state, where they require additional data including physicochemical and physiological balances and bounds (mass and energy conversion) [91]. Modeling and simulation have been widely used in several chronic

Database	Description	URL	Reference
BioCarta	A pathway database that provides gene interaction within pathways for human cellular processes	https://cgap.nci.nih.gov/Pathways/BioCarta_Pathways	[79]
HumanCyc	One of the pathway databases in BioCyc that consists of human metabolic pathways	https://humancyc.org/	[81]
Kyoto Encyclopedia of Genes and Genomes (KEGG)	A repository to understand the high-level functions and utilities of the biological system of several organisms including humans that were obtained from genome sequencing and other high-throughput experimental technologies	https://www.kegg.jp/	[80]
PANTHER	Contains several biological information such as pathways of proteins coupled with tools for protein analysis for several organisms including humans	http://pantherdb.org/	[82]
Reactome	A pathway database for several organisms including humans that provides tools for pathway analysis	https://reactome.org/	[83]
Wikipathways	A pathway database that contains pathway information of several organisms such as humans	https://www.wikipathways.org/index.php/WikiPathways	[77]

Table 2.
Lists of human pathway database.

diseases such as diabetes, Alzheimer's disease, coronary heart disease, and infectious diseases such as meningitis and influenza [89, 92–95].

In this approach, there are several types of models that have been applied to understand the human diseases, which are pharmacokinetics (PK) model, pharmacokinetics/pharmacodynamics (PKPD) model, disease progression model, metamodel, and Bayesian model averaging [90]. PK model is widely used in the field of clinical pharmacology as it simulates the rate and extent of drug distribution to different tissues and the rate and impact of drug disposition. It is a very important model as it predicts the impact variability in target patient populations in response to drug administration [96]. PKPD model is another model in the drug development where it integrates PK and PD components. This model establishes and measures the relationships of dose-concentration-response and describes and predicts the effect-time courses in consequence of a drug dose [97]. Meanwhile, the disease progression model is the time course quantitative descriptor of disease status. It was first simulated in 1992 in Alzheimer's disease using the cognitive component of the Alzheimer's disease assessment scale (ADASC) to assess the disease severity [93]. This model characterizes the natural progression of the disease by incorporating biomarkers of disease severity and/or clinical outcomes. Disease progression model is often used to quantify the effects of drug treatment on disease progression by integrating with PK and PKPD models [98]. Metamodel involves model development by combining results from multiple previous studies. In human disease study, this model can be used to compare the effects and safety of new treatments with other treatments, to reevaluate data of mixed or different result situations, and to describe PD or disease progress models [90, 99]. In the meantime, Bayesian model averaging combines models as there is a situation where previous studies show several models for a drug in a certain disease, and it is unclear which model is suitable. The Bayesian model averaging reduces the uncertainty by allowing all existing models to contribute to a simulation with weighing the inputs on the basis of certain criteria such as the quality of data or model [90, 92].

Complex diseases involve many genes, proteins, and metabolites, and these molecules are either activated or deactivated in certain tissues in particular time, depending on the disease status or in the influences of several factors such as drug administration. Hence, modeling and simulation are efficient approaches in the computational systems analysis as these approaches manage to dynamically monitor and understand the progress of diseases in particular situation, which in turn can assist in improving the specific treatment and developing the efficient drugs for complex human diseases.

4. Data repository

Data are the most important resource in computational systems analysis. Most of the analyses require the integration of several data to understand the diseases, particularly complex diseases in a systemic view. For example, several omics data (genomics, transcriptomics, proteomics, and/or metabolomics) were integrated with interactions data (PPI or pathway) to construct network biology. Modeling and simulation also involve omics data integration to capture the complexity of molecular events causing the diseases. In addition, cellular and physiological processes are complex systems [100] that are controlled by signals from the extracellular environment and coordinated by intracellular interaction and transcriptional or gene regulatory networks assembled into functional modules [101]. In order to understand cellular processes as interconnected and interdependent systems and in the context of a biological phenomenon, requires an integrative approach that draws upon data from as many diverse data sources as possible including data from the literature, public databases, biochemical and kinetic experiments, phenotype studies and high-throughput analyses of the genome, transcriptome, proteome, interactome, and metabolome.

Hence, data repository or database development is one of the main approaches to facilitate the arbitrary querying of the data to perform the computational systems analysis. Besides, recent developments in high-throughput approaches enable the analysis of the transcriptome, proteome, interactome, metabolome, and phenome on a previously unprecedented scale, thus contributing to the deluge of experimental data and scattering in an unorganized way. The data repository is one of the efforts in combining the growing sets of experimental data in a proper way that can be publicly accessed to have further analysis. For example, there are databases such as ArrayExpress [102], Gene Expression Omnibus (GEO) [103], and CIBEX [104] that stores datasets for gene expression studies to be publicly accessed. Other than that, there are also literature databases such as PubMed, Scopus Online, and Google Scholar for the researchers to retrieve published studies, and there are several studies that provide the generated omics datasets in the supplementary section.

There are also databases such as disease databases that have performed several analyses prior to deposit the data into the database. The human disease databases have been developed in order to store information about diseases such as genes, proteins, metabolites, drugs, literature, biological processes, tissues, and others that are related to a particular disease in order to understand the pathobiology, pathogenesis, and pathophysiology of diseases. Currently, databases, such as DisGeNET [105], MalaCards [106], Online Mendelian Inheritance in Man (OMIM) [51], Open Targets [107], GWAS Catalog [108], GWASdb [109], DISEASES [110], and Human Gene Mutation Database (HGMD) [111], have been developed to store several information about human diseases. There are also databases that have been developed that specifically store data or information of a disease such as T2D-Db [112] and T2D@ZJU [113] for type-2 diabetes, AlzBase [114], AlzGene [115], and NIAGADS [116] for Alzheimer's disease, and The Cancer Genome Atlas (TCGA) [117] and The International Cancer Genome Consortium (ICGC) [118] for human cancers.

Nowadays, the number of databases that hold a growing number of generated data is also increased, which has led to a new challenge in selecting the best and suitable database for further computational systems analysis. Nevertheless, the presence of current available data repository or databases has eased the researchers without having to extensively search the data to integrate the data and visualize the data into a network and/or model in order to harness a comprehensive systems-level understanding of pathophysiological processes of human diseases.

5. Computational systems analysis progress in PCOS

PCOS is a heterogeneous disorder that may be affected by multiple factors including genetic, lifestyle, and environment. The definition of PCOS is unclear, where it is defined by a combination of different features that lead to its diagnostic criteria remain controversial. PCOS women also experience multi-symptoms, and the diseases that comorbid to PCOS are widely varied [6, 119]. The complexity in PCOS is evident that many genes, proteins, and metabolites involved in the pathobiology of PCOS. All omics platforms have been applied to identifying the molecular basis of PCOS (**Table 3**) [120].

Even though all omics have been performed in PCOS, the pathobiology of PCOS is still far from understood. Since the prevalence of PCOS women is increased and if they are left untreated, PCOS women are at higher risk to develop other

Omics	Description	Examples of previous studies	Reference
Genomics	Identification genetics evidence in PCOS women	Identified 16 loci associated risk of PCOS in Chinese and European subjects	[121–124]
Transcriptomics	Identification of differentially expressed genes (significantly up-regulated and down-regulated genes) between non-PCOS and PCOS women	Identified 243 differential expressed gene in the granulosa cells between non-PCOS and PCOS patients	[125]
Proteomics	Detection of differentially expressed protein between non-PCOS and PCOS women	Identified 186 significantly expressed proteins in the follicular fluid between non-PCOS and PCOS women	[126]
Metabolomics	Detection of altered metabolites between non-PCOS and PCOS women	The altered metabolites in the sera between non-PCOS and PCOS women revealed disruptions in several metabolic pathways such as steroid hormone biosynthesis, amino acids and nucleotides metabolism, and glutathione metabolism, as well as lipids and carbohydrates metabolism	[127]

Table 3.
Omics approaches in PCOS.

chronic diseases (endometrial cancer, type-2 diabetes and cardiovascular diseases), and other approaches such as computational systems analysis need to be done to improve the understanding in PCOS. By far, several studies have integrated the omics platforms using computational systems analysis to provide a systems-level understanding of PCOS.

5.1 PPI and pathway analysis

In PCOS, PPI- and pathway-based analysis is also often used to identify the genes/proteins, ontologies, and pathways that might be involved in this disorder. Among the earliest full-paper study in using PPI analysis in PCOS was published in 2009. In this work, Mohamed-Hussein and Harun combined seven microarray datasets and integrated with PPI information and successfully identified a hypothetical protein, C1ORF123, and several ontologies that might be highly involved in PCOS [128]. Prior to this study, there is an article outline in 2007 by Menke et al. that used a Newman algorithm to identify the small set of modules in the constructed PCOS PPI network that could lead to PCOS phenotypes [129]. Shen et al. [130] have constructed the regulatory network and PPI network by integrating several data such as genome-wide methylated DNA immunoprecipitation (MeDIP), regulatory interactions and PPI to investigate the relationship of insulin resistance (IR) with PCOS. In a regulatory network, the significant methylated genes, CCAAT enhancer binding protein beta (CEBPB) formed a network that regulated other genes that may play a role in both IR and PCOS. Meanwhile, the constructed PPI network showed that the methylated genes in PCOS-IR have a higher number of interactions and might act as key drivers to perform proper cellular functions. Shen et al. [130] also found several enriched pathways such as cancer pathways and MAPK signaling and ontologies including regulation of metabolic process from both constructed networks that might be responsible in both PCOS and IR [130]. Shim et al. used pathway-based analysis on genome-wide association study (GWAS) dataset of PCOS and successfully identified several PCOS pathways associated with ovulation and insulin secretion [131].

Kori et al. [132] used PPI and pathway analysis by integrating three microarray datasets of PCOS with PPI data, performing the pathway enrichment analysis and comparing the PCOS results with ovarian cancer and endometriosis. These analyses found that PCOS is closely related to endometriosis and ovarian cancer as they shared several molecules and pathways such as MAPK signaling, cell cycle, and apoptosis [132]. The integration of a microarray dataset with PPI information from REACTOME has found several proteins including Rho GTPase activating protein 4 (ARHGAP4), Rho GTPase activating protein 9 (ARHGAP9), ras homolog family member G (RHOG) and LYN proto-oncogene, Src family tyrosine kinase (LYN), and pathways such as RhoA-related pathways, and glycoprotein VI-mediated activation cascade might involve in the PCOS pathogenesis [133].

Other than identifying the molecular basis and the biological functions that might relate to PCOS, PPI and pathway analysis are also applied to decipher the molecular relationship of PCOS with other diseases and improve the knowledge on PCOS treatments. Liu et al. [134] construct a PPI network, which consists of PCOS-related genes and target genes of Erxian decoction (EXD) to understand the pharmacological basis of the EXD action in treating PCOS. EXD is a traditional Chinese medicine composed of six types of herbs that can alleviate several problems such as ovarian failure, which is a problem that commonly experiences by PCOS women. In the constructed network, Liu et al. [134] identified 50 genes that might be key genes that involved in PCOS treatment with EXD since these genes are the EXD targets that are found to be related to PCOS [134]. Ramly et al. [135] also used PPI and pathway analysis to identify protein and pathways to explain the relationships between PCOS and 17 diseases such as migraine, ovarian cancer, and schizophrenia. They used a clustering approach by MCODE [66] to identify shared proteins between PCOS and other diseases and pathway enrichment analysis to identify pathways that might connect PCOS and PCOS-associated diseases [135].

Based on aforementioned studies, it is proved that PPI- and pathway-based can be used to identify genes/proteins, biomarkers, ontologies, and pathways that are related to PCOS, which in turn could improve the diagnosis and treatment in PCOS.

5.2 Data repository in PCOS

As mentioned, there are many datasets that have been generated by the omics platforms to identify the pathobiology of PCOS. The datasets are randomly distributed, and it is very tedious if the researchers intend to retrieve the information about PCOS. Hence, it is essential to have a repository that stores comprehensive information on PCOS.

There are three databases that have been developed by far to deposit the collated molecular information generated by previous studies, which are PCOSBase (www.pcosbase.org) [136], PCOSKB (http://pcoskb.bicnirrh.res.in/) [137], and PCOSDB (http://pcosdb.net/) [138]. Both PCOSKB and PCOSDB contain 241 and 208 genes that related to PCOS, respectively. These databases searched for the PCOS-related genes against scientific literature. Meanwhile, PCOSBase identified 8185 PCOS-related proteins that were obtained from previous disease databases and gene and protein expression studies. All of the PCOS databases provided detailed description for each entry that is related to PCOS and link to the original databases such as UniProt (https://www.uniprot.org/) and NCBI (https://www.ncbi.nlm.nih.gov/) for extensive information. As PCOSBase, biological information such as chromosomal location, gene ontologies, pathways, domains, disease-associated, and tissue localization have been annotated to all PCOS-related proteins. **Figure 5** shows the

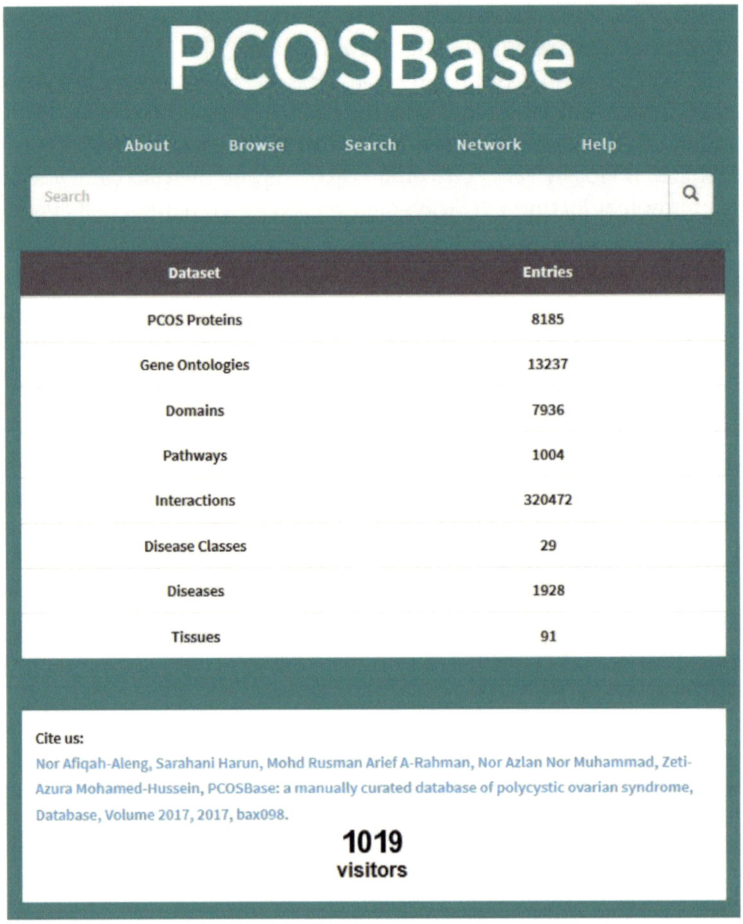

Figure 5.
PCOSBase homepage.

example homepage of PCOSBase, where it provides search box to facilitate the users to search with keywords and shows the number of entries for each functional details that are deposited in the database.

All of these databases are developed as an effort for other researchers in identifying PCOS biomarkers. Besides, the information from the databases has been used to integrate with other information such as PPI and pathway to have a systems-level view of PCOS. PCOSBase provided a menu ("Network") that contained a biological network of PCOS as examples of analysis on the PCOS-related proteins from this database. The network provided in the database can give an insight into improving the knowledge, particularly in PCOS.

6. Conclusion and future perspective

PCOS is an endocrine disorder that linked many clinical symptoms and the diversity of diseases. The PCOS complexity requires the development of novel analysis methods such as the simultaneous analysis of omics data using computational systems analysis. In addition, the availability of multi-omics datasets has opened the avenue to gain new insights into related molecular pathophysiological changes in PCOS. Thus, the previously generated data should be fully utilized as a whole to have a systems-view of PCOS. As mentioned in this chapter, the computation systems analysis such as PPI and pathway analysis has been performed, and several examples of studies using this approach have been provided. The specific data repository of PCOS has also been developed, which could be used for further analysis by PCOS researchers. However, there is a lack of studies that integrate the omics datasets using modeling and simulation to investigate PCOS in a systems-level. This approach should be put into consideration in the future as this approach can dynamically elucidate the PCOS progression and improve the PCOS diagnosis and treatment. Although there is a limitation particularly the state of the incompleteness of biological information such as human interactome and pathway annotation, the analysis on current data by computational systems analysis should be continuously performed as these efforts could constantly enhance the knowledge of a complex syndrome, which is PCOS.

Acknowledgements

This research was supported by the Ministry of Higher Education, Malaysia, (FRGS/1/2014/SGD5/UKM/02/6) and Universiti Kebangsaan Malaysia (grant DIP2018-004). N.A.-A.'s Ph.D. scholarship is funded by the MyBrain15 program from the Ministry of Higher Education, Malaysia.

Conflict of interest

The authors declare no conflict of interest.

Author details

Nor Afiqah-Aleng[1,2] and Zeti-Azura Mohamed-Hussein[1,3]*

1 Centre for Bioinformatics Research, Institute of Systems Biology (INBIOSIS), Universiti Kebangsaan Malaysia (UKM), Bangi, Selangor, Malaysia

2 Institute of Marine Biotechnology, Universiti Malaysia Terengganu (UMT), Terengganu, Malaysia

3 Centre for Frontier Sciences, Faculty of Science and Technology, Universiti Kebangsaan Malaysia (UKM), Bangi, Selangor, Malaysia

*Address all correspondence to: zeti.hussein@ukm.edu.my

References

[1] Chakravorty S, Williams TN. Sickle cell disease: A neglected chronic disease of increasing global health importance. Archives of Disease in Childhood. 2015;**100**:48-53

[2] Mannucci P, Tuddenham E. The hemophilias—From royal genes to gene therapy. The New England Journal of Medicine. 2001;**344**:1773-1779

[3] Davidson DJ, Porteous DJ. The genetics of cystic fibrosis lung disease. Thorax. 1998;**53**:389-397

[4] Kharroubi AT, Darwish HM. Diabetes mellitus: The epidemic of the century. World Journal of Diabetes. 2015;**6**:850-867

[5] Lara-Pezzi E, Dopazo A, Manzanares M. Understanding cardiovascular disease: A journey through the genome (and what we found there). Disease Models & Mechanisms. 2012;**5**:434-443

[6] Escobar-Morreale HF. Polycystic ovary syndrome: Definition, aetiology, diagnosis and treatment. Nature Reviews. Endocrinology. 2018;**14**:270-284

[7] Rutter H. The complex systems challenge of obesity. Clinical Chemistry. 2018;**64**:44-46

[8] Gonzalez MW, Kann MG. Protein interactions and disease. PLoS Computational Biology. 2012;**8**:e1002819

[9] Barabási AL, Oltvai ZN. Network biology: Understanding the cell's functional organization. Nature Reviews Genetics. 2004;**5**:101-113

[10] Barabási A-L, Gulbahce N, Loscalzo J. Network medicine: A network-based approach to human disease. Nature Reviews Genetics. 2011;**12**:56-68

[11] Safari-Alighiarloo N, Taghizadeh M, Rezaei-Tavirani M, et al. Protein-protein interaction networks (PPI) and complex diseases. Gastroenterology and Hepatology From Bed to Bench. 2014;**7**:17-31

[12] Milo R. What is the total number of protein molecules per cell volume? A call to rethink some published values. BioEssays. 2013;**35**:1050-1055

[13] Sevimoglu T, Arga KY. The role of protein interaction networks in systems biomedicine. Computational and Structural Biotechnology Journal. 2014;**11**:22-27

[14] Chuang H-Y, Lee E, Liu Y-T, et al. Network-based classification of breast cancer metastasis. Molecular Systems Biology. 2007;**3**:140

[15] Bergholdt R, Brorsson C, Palleja A, et al. Identification of novel type 1 diabetes candidate genes by integrating genome-wide association data, protein-protein interactions, and human pancreatic islet gene expression. Diabetes. 2012;**61**:954-962

[16] Tourette C, Li B, Bell R, et al. A large scale huntingtin protein interaction network implicates RHO GTPase signaling pathways in Huntington disease. The Journal of Biological Chemistry. 2014;**289**:6709-6726

[17] Ito T, Chiba T, Ozawa R, et al. A comprehensive two-hybrid analysis to explore the yeast protein interactome. Proceedings of the National Academy of Sciences. 2001;**98**:4569-4574

[18] Uetz P, Giot L, Cagney G, et al. A comprehensive analysis of protein-protein interactions in *Saccharomyces cerevisiae*. Nature. 2000;**403**:623-627

[19] Gavin AC, Aloy P, Grandi P, et al. Proteome survey reveals modularity

of the yeast cell machinery. Nature. 2006;**440**:631-636

[20] Krogan NJ, Cagney G, Yu H, et al. Global landscape of protein complexes in the yeast *Saccharomyces cerevisiae*. Nature. 2006;**440**:637-643

[21] Fossum E, Friedel CC, Rajagopala SV, et al. Evolutionarily conserved herpesviral protein interaction networks. PLoS Pathogens. 2009;**5**:e1000570

[22] Peregrín-Alvarez JM, Xiong X, Su C, et al. The modular organization of protein interactions in *Escherichia coli*. PLoS Computational Biology. 2009;**5**:e1000523

[23] Li S, Armstrong CM, Bertin N, et al. A map of the interactome network of the metazoan *C. elegans*. Science. 2004;**303**:540-543

[24] Giot L, Bader JS, Brouwer C, et al. A protein interaction map of *Drosophila melanogaster*. Science. 2003;**302**:1727-1736

[25] Rual JF, Venkatesan K, Hao T, et al. Towards a proteome-scale map of the human protein-protein interaction network. Nature. 2005;**437**:1173-1178

[26] Stelzl U, Worm U, Lalowski M, et al. A human protein-protein interaction network: A resource for annotating the proteome. Cell. 2005;**122**:957-968

[27] Stark C, Breitkreutz B-J, Reguly T, et al. BioGRID: A general repository for interaction datasets. Nucleic Acids Research. 2006;**34**:D535-D539

[28] Salwinski L, Miller CS, Smith AJ, et al. The database of interacting proteins: 2004 update. Nucleic Acids Research. 2004;**32**:D449-D451

[29] Franz M, Rodriguez H, Lopes C, et al. GeneMANIA update 2018. Nucleic Acids Research. 2018;**46**:W60-W64

[30] Alanis-Lobato G, Andrade-Navarro MA, Schaefer MH. HIPPIE v2.0: Enhancing meaningfulness and reliability of protein-protein interaction networks. Nucleic Acids Research. 2017;**45**:D408-D414

[31] Prasad KS, Goel R, Kandasamy K, et al. Human protein reference database—2009 update. Nucleic Acids Research. 2009;**37**:D767-D772

[32] Brown KR, Jurisica I. Unequal evolutionary conservation of human protein interactions in interologous networks. Genome Biology. 2007;**8**:R95

[33] Orchard S, Ammari M, Aranda B, et al. The MIntAct project—IntAct as a common curation platform for 11 molecular interaction databases. Nucleic Acids Research. 2014;**42**:D358-D363

[34] Pagel P, Kovac S, Oesterheld M, et al. The MIPS mammalian protein-protein interaction database. Bioinformatics. 2005;**21**:832-834

[35] Chatr-aryamontri A, Ceol A, Palazzi LM, et al. The molecular interaction database. Nucleic Acids Research. 2007;**35**:D572-D574

[36] Szklarczyk D, Morris JH, Cook H, et al. The STRING database in 2017: Quality-controlled protein-protein association networks, made broadly accessible. Nucleic Acids Research. 2017;**45**:D362-D368

[37] Alonso-López D, Campos-Laborie FJ, Gutiérrez MA, et al. APID database: redefining protein-protein interaction experimental evidences and binary interactomes. Database. 2019;**2019**:baz005

[38] Xenarios I. DIP: The database of interacting proteins: 2001 update. Nucleic Acids Research. 2001;**29**:289-291

[39] Hoffmann R, Valencia A. A gene network for navigating the literature. Nature Genetics. 2004;**36**:664

[40] Breuer K, Foroushani AK, Laird MR, et al. InnateDB: Systems biology of innate immunity and beyond—Recent updates and continuing curation. Nucleic Acids Research. 2013;**41**:D1228-D1233

[41] Licata L, Briganti L, Peluso D, et al. The molecular interaction database: 2012 update. Nucleic Acids Research. 2012;**40**:D857-D861

[42] Launay G, Salza R, Multedo D, et al. MatrixDB, the extracellular matrix interaction database: Updated content, a new navigator and expanded functionalities. Nucleic Acids Research. 2015;**43**:D321-D327

[43] Han K, Park B, Kim H, et al. HPID: The human protein interaction. Bioinformatics. 2004;**20**:2466-2470

[44] Orchard S, Kerrien S, Abbani S, et al. Protein interaction data curation—The international molecular exchange consortium (IMEx). Nature Methods. 2012;**9**:345-350

[45] Kuchaiev O, Pržulj N. Integrative network alignment reveals large regions of global network similarity in yeast and human. Bioinformatics. 2011;**27**:1390-1396

[46] Memisevic V, Milenkovic T, Przulj N. Complementarity of network and sequence information in homologous proteins. Journal of Integrative Bioinformatics. 2010;**7**:135

[47] Ideker T, Sharan R. Protein networks in disease. Genome Research. 2008;**18**:644-652

[48] Liu W, Wu A, Pellegrini M, et al. Integrative analysis of human protein, function and disease networks. Scientific Reports. 2015;**5**:14344

[49] Wachi S, Yoneda K, Wu R. Interactome-transcriptome analysis reveals the high centrality of genes differentially expressed in lung cancer tissues. Bioinformatics. 2005;**21**:4205-4208

[50] Jonsson PF, Bates PA. Global topological features of cancer proteins in the human interactome. Bioinformatics. 2006;**22**:2291-2297

[51] Amberger JS, Bocchini CA, Schiettecatte F, et al. OMIM.org: Online mendelian inheritance in man (OMIM®), an online catalog of human genes and genetic disorders. Nucleic Acids Research. 2015;**43**:D789-D798

[52] Krauthammer M, Kaufmann CA, Gilliam TC, et al. Molecular triangulation: Bridging linkage and molecular-network information for identifying candidate genes in Alzheimer's disease. Proceedings of the National Academy of Sciences. 2004;**101**:15148-15153

[53] Oti M, Snel B, Huynen MA, et al. Predicting disease genes using protein-protein interactions. Journal of Medical Genetics. 2006;**43**:691-698

[54] Navlakha S, Kingsford C. The power of protein interaction networks for associating genes with diseases. Bioinformatics. 2010;**26**:1057-1063

[55] Adamcsek B, Palla G, Farkas IJ, et al. CFinder: Locating cliques and overlapping modules in biological networks. Bioinformatics. 2006;**22**:1021-1023

[56] Nepusz T, Yu H, Paccanaro A. Detecting overlapping protein complexes in protein-protein interaction networks. Nature Methods. 2012;**9**:471-472

[57] Liu G, Wong L, Chua HN. Complex discovery from weighted PPI networks. Bioinformatics. 2009;**25**:1891-1897

[58] Palla G, Derényi I, Farkas I, et al. Uncovering the overlapping community structure of complex networks in nature and society. Nature. 2005;**435**:814-818

[59] Altaf-Ul-Amin M, Shinbo Y, Mihara K, et al. Development and implementation of an algorithm for detection of protein complexes in large interaction networks. BMC Bioinformatics. 2006;**7**:207

[60] Altaf-Ul-Amin M, Wada M, Kanaya S. Partitioning a PPI network into overlapping modules constrained by high-density and periphery tracking. ISRN Biomathematics. 2012;**2012**:726429

[61] Mohammad BK, Wakamatsu N, Md A-U-A. DPClusOST: A software tool for general purpose graph clustering. Journal of Computer Aided Chemistry. 2017;**18**:76-93

[62] Li M, Chen JE, Wang JX, et al. Modifying the DPClus algorithm for identifying protein complexes based on new topological structures. BMC Bioinformatics. 2008;**9**:398

[63] Li X-L, Tan S-H, Foo C-S, et al. Interaction graph mining for protein complexes using local clique merging. Genome Informatics: International Conference on Genome Informatics. 2005;**16**:260-269

[64] King AD, Pržulj N, Jurisica I. Protein complex prediction via cost-based clustering. Bioinformatics. 2004;**20**:3013-3020

[65] Enright AJ, Van Dongen S, Ouzounis CA. An efficient algorithm for large-scale detection of protein families. Nucleic Acids Research. 2002;**30**:1575-1584

[66] Bader GD, Hogue CWV. An automated method for finding molecular complexes in large protein interaction networks. BMC Bioinformatics. 2003;**4**:2

[67] Wu X, Jiang R, Zhang MQ, et al. Network-based global inference of human disease genes. Molecular Systems Biology. 2008;**4**:189

[68] Rezaei-Tavirani M, Rezaei-Tavirani S, Mansouri V, et al. Protein-protein interaction network analysis for a biomarker panel related to human esophageal adenocarcinoma. Asian Pacific Journal of Cancer Prevention. 2017;**18**:3357-3363

[69] Xiao H, Yang L, Liu J, et al. Protein-protein interaction analysis to identify biomarker networks for endometriosis. Experimental and Therapeutic Medicine. 2017;**14**:4647-4654

[70] Hidalgo CA, Blumm N, Barabási AL, et al. A dynamic network approach for the study of human phenotypes. PLoS Computational Biology. 2009;**5**:e1000353

[71] Sun K, Gonçalves JP, Larminie C, et al. Predicting disease associations via biological network analysis. BMC Bioinformatics. 2014;**15**:304

[72] Ko Y, Cho M, Lee JS, et al. Identification of disease comorbidity through hidden molecular mechanisms. Scientific Reports. 2016;**6**:39433

[73] Goh K-I, Cusick ME, Valle D, et al. The human disease network. Proceedings of the National Academy of Sciences. 2007;**104**:8685-8690

[74] Ahmed SS, Ahameethunisa AR, Santosh W, et al. Systems biological approach on neurological disorders: A novel molecular connectivity to aging and psychiatric diseases. BMC Systems Biology. 2011;**5**:6

[75] Kanehisa M, Sato Y, Kawashima M, et al. KEGG as a reference resource for gene and protein annotation. Nucleic Acids Research. 2016;**44**:D457-D462

[76] Croft D, O'Kelly G, Wu G, et al. Reactome: A database of reactions,

pathways and biological processes. Nucleic Acids Research. 2011;**39**:D691-D697

[77] Pico AR, Kelder T, Van Iersel MP, et al. WikiPathways: Pathway editing for the people. PLoS Biology. 2008;**6**:e184

[78] Karp PD, Billington R, Caspi R, et al. The BioCyc collection of microbial genomes and metabolic pathways. Briefings in Bioinformatics. 2017;**2017**:bbx085

[79] Nishimura D. A view from the web. BioCarta. Biotech Software & Internet Report. 2001;**2**:117-120

[80] Kanehisa M, Furumichi M, Tanabe M, et al. KEGG: New perspectives on genomes, pathways, diseases and drugs. Nucleic Acids Research. 2016;**45**:353-361

[81] Trupp M, Altman T, Fulcher CA, et al. Beyond the genome (BTG) is a (PGDB) pathway genome database: HumanCyc. Genome Biology. 2010;**11**:O12

[82] Mi H, Thomas P. PANTHER pathway: An ontology-based pathway database coupled with data analysis tools. Methods in Molecular Biology. 2009;**563**:123-140

[83] Fabregat A, Jupe S, Matthews L, et al. The reactome pathway knowledgebase. Nucleic Acids Research. 2018;**46**:D649-D655

[84] Torres-Ayuso P, Sahoo S, Ashton G, et al. Signaling pathway screening platforms are an efficient approach to identify therapeutic targets in cancers that lack known driver mutations: A case report for a cancer of unknown primary origin. NPJ Genomic Medicine. 2018;**3**:15

[85] Sebastian-Leon P, Vidal E, Minguez P, et al. Understanding disease mechanisms with models of signaling pathway activities. BMC Systems Biology. 2014;**8**:121

[86] Varala K, Marshall-Colón A, Cirrone J, et al. Temporal transcriptional logic of dynamic regulatory networks underlying nitrogen signaling and use in plants. Proceedings of the National Academy of Sciences of the United States of America. 2018;**115**:6494-6499

[87] Doong SJ, Gupta A, Prather KLJ. Layered dynamic regulation for improving metabolic pathway productivity in *Escherichia coli*. Proceedings of the National Academy of Sciences. 2018;**115**:2964-2969

[88] Alaimo S, Marceca G, Ferro A, et al. Detecting disease specific pathway substructures through an integrated systems biology approach. Non-Coding RNA. 2017;**3**:20

[89] Barhak J, Isaman DJ, Ye W, et al. Chronic disease modeling and simulation software. Journal of Biomedical Informatics. 2010;**43**:791-799

[90] Mould D, Upton R. Basic concepts in population modeling, simulation, and model-based drug development. CPT: Pharmacometrics & Systems Pharmacology. 2012;**1**:e6

[91] Edwards LM, Thiele I. Appling systems biology methods to the study of human physiology in extreme environment. Extreme Physiology & Medicine. 2013;**2**:8

[92] Wang D, Lertsithichai P, Nanchahal K, et al. Risk factors of coronary heart disease: A Bayesian model averaging approach. Journal of Applied Statistics. 2003;**30**:813-826

[93] Holford NH, Peace KE. Results and validation of a population pharmacodynamic model for cognitive effects in Alzheimer patients treated with tacrine. Proceedings of the

National Academy of Sciences. 1992;**89**:11471-11475

[94] Gambhir M, Bozio C, O'Hagan JJ, et al. Infectious disease modeling methods as tools for informing response to novel influenza viruses of unknown pandemic potential. Clinical Infectious Diseases. 2015;**60**:S11-S19

[95] Jackson ML, Diallo AO, Médah I, et al. Initial validation of a simulation model for estimating the impact of serogroup A Neisseria meningitidis vaccination in the African meningitis belt. PLoS One. 2018;**13**:e0206117

[96] Kiang TKL, Sherwin CMT, Spigarelli MG, et al. Fundamentals of population pharmacokinetic modelling. Clinical Pharmacokinetics. 2015;**51**:515-525

[97] Meibohm B, Derendorf H. Basic concepts of pharmacokinetic/pharmacodynamic (PK/PD) modelling. International Journal of Clinical Pharmacology and Therapeutics. 1997;**35**:401-413

[98] Cook SF, Bies RR. Disease progression modeling: Key concepts and recent developments. Current Pharmacology Reports. 2016;**2**:221-230

[99] Burke DS, Grefenstette JJ. Toward an integrated meta-model of public health dynamics for preparedness decision support. Journal of Public Health Management and Practice. 2013;**19**:S12-S15

[100] Kitano H. Computational systems biology. Nature. 2002;**420**:206-210

[101] Hartwell LH, Hopfield JJ, Leibler S, et al. From molecular to modular cell biology. Nature. 1999;**402**:C47-C52

[102] Kolesnikov N, Hastings E, Keays M, et al. Array express update-simplifying data submissions. Nucleic Acids Research. 2015;**43**:D1113-D1116

[103] Clough E, Barrett T. The gene expression omnibus database. Methods in Molecular Biology. 2016;**1418**:93-110

[104] Ikeo K, Ishi-i J, Tamura T, et al. CIBEX: Center for information biology gene expression database. Comptes Rendus Biologies. 2003;**326**:1079-1082

[105] Pinero J, Bravo A, Queralt-Rosinach N, et al. DisGeNET: A comprehensive platform integrating information on human disease-associated genes and variants. Nucleic Acids Research. 2017;**45**:D833-D839

[106] Rappaport N, Twik M, Plaschkes I, et al. MalaCards: An amalgamated human disease compendium with diverse clinical and genetic annotation and structured search. Nucleic Acids Research. 2017;**45**:D877-D887

[107] Carvalho-Silva D, Pierleoni A, Pignatelli M, et al. Open targets platform: New developments and updates two years on. Nucleic Acids Research. 2019;**47**:D1056-D1065

[108] Welter D, MacArthur J, Morales J, et al. The NHGRI GWAS catalog, a curated resource of SNP-trait associations. Nucleic Acids Research. 2014;**42**:D1001-D1006

[109] Li MJ, Liu Z, Wang P, et al. GWASdb v2: An update database for human genetic variants identified by genome-wide association studies. Nucleic Acids Research. 2016;**44**:D869-D876

[110] Pletscher-Frankild S, Pallejà A, Tsafou K, et al. DISEASES: Text mining and data integration of disease-gene associations. Methods. 2015;**74**:83-89

[111] Stenson PD, Mort M, Ball EV, et al. The human gene mutation database: Towards a comprehensive repository of inherited mutation data for medical research, genetic diagnosis and

next-generation sequencing studies. Human Genetics. 2017;**136**:665-677

[112] Agrawal S, Dimitrova N, Nathan P, et al. T2D-Db: An integrated platform to study the molecular basis of type 2 diabetes. BMC Genomics. 2008;**9**:320

[113] Yang Z, Yang J, Liu W, et al. T2D@ZJU: A knowledgebase integrating heterogeneous connections associated with type 2 diabetes mellitus. Database. 2013;**2013**:bat052

[114] Bai Z, Han G, Xie B, et al. AlzBase: An integrative database for Ggene dysregulation in Alzheimer's disease. Molecular Neurobiology. 2016;**53**:310-319

[115] Nia BV, Kang C, Tran MG, et al. Meta analysis of human AlzGene database: Benefits and limitations of using C. elegans for the study of Alzheimer's disease and co-morbid conditions. Frontiers in Genetics. 2017;**8**:55

[116] Kuzma A, Valladares O, Cweibel R, et al. NIAGADS: The NIA genetics of Alzheimer's disease data storage site. Alzheimer's & Dementia. 2016;**12**:1200-1203

[117] Hutter C, Zenklusen JC. The cancer genome atlas: Creating lasting value beyond its data. Cell. 2018;**173**:283-285

[118] Zhang J, Baran J, Cros A, et al. International cancer genome consortium data portal-a one-stop shop for cancer genomics data. Database. 2011;**2011**:bar026

[119] Azziz R, Carmina E, Chen Z, et al. Polycystic ovary syndrome. Nature Reviews Disease Primers. 2016;**2**:16057

[120] Afiqah-Aleng N, Mohamed-Hussein ZA. Computational systems biology approach on polycystic ovarian syndrome (PCOS). Journal of Molecular and Genetic Medicine. 2019;**13**:1000392

[121] Chen Z-J, Zhao H, He L, et al. Genome-wide association study identifies susceptibility loci for polycystic ovary syndrome on chromosome 2p16.3, 2p21 and 9q33.3. Nature Genetics. 2011;**43**:55-59

[122] Shi Y, Zhao H, Shi Y, et al. Genome-wide association study identifies eight new risk loci for polycystic ovary syndrome. Nature Genetics. 2012;**44**:1020-1025

[123] Hayes MG, Urbanek M, Ehrmann DA, et al. Genome-wide association of polycystic ovary syndrome implicates alterations in gonadotropin secretion in European ancestry populations. Nature Communications. 2015;**6**:1-12

[124] Day FR, Hinds DA, Tung JY, et al. Causal mechanisms and balancing selection inferred from genetic associations with polycystic ovary syndrome. Nature Communications. 2015;**6**:8464

[125] Lan C-W, Chen M-J, Tai K-Y, et al. Functional microarray analysis of differentially expressed genes in granulosa cells from women with polycystic ovary syndrome related to MAPK/ERK signaling. Scientific Reports. 2015;**5**:14994

[126] Ambekar AS, Kelkar DS, Pinto SM, et al. Proteomics of follicular fluid from women with polycystic ovary syndrome suggests molecular defects in follicular development. The Journal of Clinical Endocrinology and Metabolism. 2015;**100**:744-753

[127] Dong F, Deng D, Chen H, et al. Serum metabolomics study of polycystic ovary syndrome based on UPLC-QTOF-MS coupled with a pattern recognition approach. Analytical and Bioanalytical Chemistry. 2015;**407**:4683-4695

[128] Mohamed-Hussein ZA, Harun S. Construction of a polycystic ovarian

syndrome (PCOS) pathway based on the interactions of PCOS-related proteins retrieved from bibliomic data. Theoretical Biology and Medical Modelling. 2009;**6**:18

[129] Menke NB, Bonchev DG, Witten TM, et al. A novel computational approach to the genetics of polycystic ovarian syndrome (PCOS). Fertility and Sterility. 2007;**88**:S73

[130] Shen H, Qiu L, Zhang Z, et al. Genome-wide methylated DNA immunoprecipitation analysis of patients with polycystic ovary syndrome. PLoS One. 2013;**8**:e64801

[131] Shim U, Kim HN, Lee H, et al. Pathway analysis based on a genome-wide association study of polycystic ovary syndrome. PLoS One. 2015;**10**:e0136609

[132] Kori M, Gov E, Arga KY. Molecular signatures of ovarian diseases: Insights from network medicine perspective. Systems Biology in Reproductive Medicine. 2016;**62**:266-282

[133] Shen H, Liang Z, Zheng S, et al. Pathway and network-based analysis of genome-wide association studies and RT-PCR validation in polycystic ovary syndrome. International Journal of Molecular Medicine. 2017;**40**:1385-1396

[134] Liu L, Du B, Zhang H, et al. A network pharmacology approach to explore the mechanisms of Erxian decoction in polycystic ovary syndrome. Chinese Medicine. 2018;**13**:46

[135] Ramly B, Afiqah-Aleng N, Mohamed-Hussein Z-A. Protein–protein interaction network analysis reveals several diseases highly associated with polycystic ovarian syndrome. International Journal of Molecular Sciences. 2019;**20**:2959

[136] Afiqah-Aleng N, Harun S, A-Rahman MR, et al. PCOSBase: A manually curated database of polycystic ovarian syndrome. Database. 2017;**2017**:bax098

[137] Joseph S, Barai RS, Bhujbalrao R, et al. PCOSKB: A knowledgebase on genes, diseases, ontology terms and biochemical pathways associated with polycystic ovary syndrome. Nucleic Acids Research. 2016;**44**:D1032-D1035

[138] Maniraja JM, Vetrivel U, Munuswamy D, et al. PCOSDB: PolyCystic ovary syndrome database for manually curated genes associated with the disease. Bioinformation. 2016;**12**:4-8